Healing Yourself During Pregnancy

Joy Gardner

The Crossing Press
Freedom, California 95019

Note to the Reader

The reader's attention is directed to the preface in which the author explains that the various treatments and other suggestions described for dealing with certain conditions, although based upon information she has gathered from the personal experiences of a number of individuals, has neither been tested on a broad sample of individuals, nor scientifically established. Therefore, neither the author nor the publisher can take responsibility for any ill effects which may be produced as a result of following any suggestions given: the reader does so at his or her own risk. The author and publisher wish to stress that the suggestions offered are based on the assumption that the condition in question has been correctly diagnosed.

Copyright © 1987 by Joy Gardner
Edited by Andrea Chesman
Cover illustration by Elayne Sears

Printed in the U.S.A. by McNaughton & Gunn of Ann Arbor, Michigan

Library of Congress Cataloging-in-Publication Data
Gardner, Joy.
    Healing yourself during pregnancy.

    Bibliography: p.
    Includes index.
    1. Pregnancy. 2. Childbirth. 3. Herbs—Therapeutic use. 4.   Naturopathy. I. Title.
[DNLM: 1. Medicine, Herbal—popular   works.   2.   Naturopathy—popular   works.
3. Pregnancy—popular works. 4. Pregnancy Complications—therapy—popular works. WQ
150 G227h]
RG525.H36   1987   613.2   87-20088
ISBN 0-89594-251-8 (pbk.)

ACKNOWLEDGMENTS

Numerous people have helped me with this book. It has been a labor of love. I particularly want to thank the following for reading parts of my manuscript and providing professional and editorial comments: Marion Toepke, nurse-practitioner and nurse-midwife; Carol Hird, R.N. and past president of the Midwives Association of British Columbia; Norman Farnsworth, Ph.D., head of the Department of Pharmacology and Pharmacognosy at the University of Illinois; Jim Campbell, M.D.; Cathrin Prince Leslie, midwife; Andrea Chesman, editor.

And thanks also to all those who answered my questionnaires and gave freely of their time and their knowledge.

Contents

Preface

I believe that we can begin and end our lives in harmony with ourselves, each other, the plants, the animals, the earth, and the cosmos. I believe that the way we come into this life and the way we depart from it set the tone for this life and the life beyond.

The use of herbs and other natural remedies enables us to maintain our connection with the earth and the plants. It is a gentle way of healing that enhances the natural harmony of the body. Pregnant women, and the babies they carry, are particularly sensitive to whatever goes into their bodies. So pregnancy is the perfect time to begin to use natural remedies.

This book is not meant to be a substitute for a doctor. Doctors are well-trained in diagnosis, and if anything is seriously wrong with you, find a doctor, midwife, naturopath, chiropractor, or other medical worker you can trust. Don't fool around with self-diagnosis. Once you know what's wrong, you may benefit from this material.

For each ailment described in this book, I have given just two or three remedies. In each case, I have chosen the remedies that have been most successful for the greatest number of people. Many of them have been tried by twenty-five to one hundred people, with favorable results. But some have been tried by as few as three. In any case, it's a scientifically small number, so if you do choose to try any remedy, *use it at your own risk.*

We are, admittedly, being our own guinea pigs. But we can be assured that most healing herbs have been a part of the human experiment for thousands of years.

Nevertheless, just because a substance is "natural" is no guarantee that it will be harmless. For example, recent studies have shown that comfrey, a very popular herb, contains cancer-causing substances. I discussed this with Norman Farnsworth, Ph.D., head of the Department of Pharmacology and Pharmacognosy at the University of Illinois. He tested many samples of comfrey roots and leaves and found small amounts of cancer-causing substances in most roots and in some leaves.

His personal opinion is that it probably would not be harmful for an adult male or nonpregnant female, for example, to drink comfrey leaf tea two or three times a week. However, in the case of a pregnant woman, even a minute amount of a possibly harmful substance could harm the fetus, so he suggests that pregnant women avoid comfrey tea entirely, though external use is all right.

xi

When I first began to learn about natural healing in 1966, I didn't know of any herbal or nutritional schools. I learned through apprenticing with herbalists and teachers of all sorts, by reading voraciously, and by experimenting on myself and on willing friends. Then I worked at a clinic as a paramedic and as a herbal and nutritional consultant, and I did careful follow-up on all my clients.

I learned by listening to anybody who would share their healing experiences. I learned from American Indians, and Italian farmers, and people from the Deep South, and the ladies at the laundromat.

Presently I work as a wholistic healer and counselor in private practice, using visualization, hypnosis, emotional release, color and gemstone therapy, toning, death and loss counseling, and even past-life regressions. Herbalism and nutrition continue to be an essential part of my practice.

Over the years I have taught in various parts of the United States and Canada, including the Victoria, B.C., Association for the Healing Arts School of Herbal Studies and Nourishment (Victoria, B.C.), Green Shores Herbal School (Vancouver, B.C.), The California School of Herbal Studies, and The Evergreen Retreat in Idaho.

In 1966 I compiled a little yellow booklet entitled *Healing Yourself*. It was published by the Country Doctor Clinic in Seattle, Washington. When I left Seattle, I continued to publish it myself. The booklet proved so useful that it sold 100,000 copies. It is available from The Crossing Press.

Healing Yourself was based on experience — my own, and the experience of those who were willing to share their knowledge with me. All of these remedies were written on index cards. Whenever someone tried one of these remedies, I would write down the results. No remedy was ever too strange for me. My main question was, "Does it really work?" And then, "Will it work again? — And again?"

Eventually all these remedies were compiled in *Healing Yourself*. Because it was one of the first contemporary books about natural healing, people from all over North America (and elsewhere) wrote to me, thanking me personally for the book. Many of these were professional and lay healers, including a large number of midwives.

Eventually I decided to do an expanded version of *Healing Yourself*. My plan for the new book was to go from birth to death, giving remedies for all the common ailments that were likely to occur. I wanted to update my information, so I prepared a list of new remedies and sent them to one hundred healers on my mailing list. I also sent a questionnaire, asking: Have you tried these remedies? Did you find them effective? If not, which remedies do you prefer?

To my amazement, fifty dedicated and generous souls answered my questionnaire. In this way, I accumulated a contemporary analysis of natural healing as it is being practiced in North America (and elsewhere).

It was fascinating to discover, for example, that shepherd's purse tea was used to prevent or stop hemorrhaging by midwives in Oregon, Indiana, British Columbia, and Mexico. And that people from Washington, Vermont, and California independently concluded that chaparrel tea as a douche for trichomonas vaginal infections worked only about 50 percent of the time. It's difficult to believe that these remedies work "just because people believe in them" when you hear so much agreement about what does and doesn't work.

Since many people who responded were midwives, I acquired an enormous volume of information on pregnancy and childbirth, which formed the basis for this book.

May you be in good health and good spirit. May you use this book to nourish yourself and to bring forth the new life within you in a good and fulfilling way.

Chapter 1
Preparing for Pregnancy

The powerful world of pregnancy holds the joy and the awe of creating a whole new person who will be a part of your life, indefinitely. When you are thinking about having a child, you may focus primarily on the nine months of pregnancy and the dramatic moment of birth. But remember that this is, literally, just the beginning: That same baby becomes terribly two, fearsomely four, delightfully six, appallingly thirteen, disturbingly twenty-eight, wonderfully thirty-two, and apprehensively forty.

A child can be the greatest gift, if you are ready for it. Becoming a parent may be the most serious choice you'll ever make. For many years, it's a twenty-four-hour-a-day job that you have the pleasure of doing when you want to, and no choice about doing when no one else wants to.

When you truly love and want your baby, it's not too difficult to wake in the middle of the night; to change endless diapers; to have less time and energy for yourself, for reading, for making love. But an unexpected or ambivalent pregnancy can bring many sorrows.

There's no commitment that two people can make that is as binding and exciting as choosing to have a baby together. It's miraculous when the love of two beings creates a third. It goes beyond any contractual agreement. You can get married and divorced and never see your partner again. But when you have a child, you will probably be a permanent part of one another's lives.

Remember that children do take after both parents, and not just physically. Your child may replicate its father (or its mother) in up to 100 percent of its characteristics. Many of your partner's personality traits, habit patterns, natural preferences, natural appetites and aptitudes (or lack of them) may show up in your child. This can happen even if the child never meets his or her father.

Whether you're a man or a woman, if you're considering having a baby and haven't found a partner, try to find someone you enjoy living with, because you'll be sharing your life with a child who closely resembles that person for a long, long time.

WANTING A BABY

Your womb is your child's first world. Because it's the first, it can make a powerful impression. Scientific research has shown that from the sixth month in utero onward, the developing baby can already remember, hear, and even learn.

Dr. Monika Lukesch, a psychologist at Constantine University in Frankfurt, West Germany, found that the mother's feelings about having a baby had the single greatest effect on an infant's physical and emotional well-being. The children of accepting mothers who looked forward to having a family were much healthier, emotionally and physically, at birth and afterward, than the offspring of rejecting mothers.

Dr. Gerhard Rottmann of the University of Salzburg, Austria, came to the same conclusion. The women who definitely wanted their babies had the easiest pregnancies, the most trouble-free births, and the healthiest offspring—physically and emotionally. The women with negative attitudes had the most devastating medical problems during pregnancy and bore the highest rate of premature, low birth weight babies. Many of these infants later showed signs of being emotionally disturbed.

But the most interesting data came from the ambivalent mothers. Some were outwardly happy about their pregnancies, but psychological testing showed that they felt ambivalent subconsciously. At birth, an unusually large number of their babies had both behavioral and gastro-intestinal problems. Another group of ambivalent mothers subconsciously wanted to be pregnant, but they were consciously in conflict because of their careers, financial problems, or their relationships. An unusually large number of these infants were apathetic or lethargic.

It seems unfair to suggest that a pregnant woman's ambivalence could have a disturbing effect on her unborn child. What pregnant woman has not experienced some ambivalence? But it is not the fleeting moments or even weeks of ambivalence that are likely to have a lasting effect—it is the persistent unreliability and unpredictability of the mother's loving energy that is terribly confusing to the unborn child, just as it is to any child.

But how can a fetus react to love or fear, when he or she has no experience of these feelings? In his book, *The Secret Life of the Unborn Child*, Dr. Thomas Verny explains that fear and anxiety can be biochemically induced by the injection of a group of chemicals called catecholamines, which appear naturally in the blood of fearful animals and humans. When these chemicals are injected into the blood of relaxed animals, they begin acting terrified within seconds. These chemicals produce all the physiological reactions we associate with fear and anxiety. It has also been shown that within a fraction of a second after the mother's heart speeds up (a common reaction to fear), the baby's heart begins pounding at double its normal rate. Understanding this helps us to appreciate how profoundly the mother's feelings influence her baby.

If you are feeling ambivalent about having a child, I don't think you should see this as a reason not to have a baby. "Behavioral and gastro-intestinal problems" could mean anything from a little colic to severe hyperactivity. "Apathetic and lethargic" could range from just sleeping a lot (things could be worse!) to severe thyroid problems. My experience has been that the severity of the mother's ambivalence is usually reflected in the severity of the child's responses.

If you feel significantly ambivalent, a good counselor may be able to help you. For example, your feelings about your own mother and your own birth are factors that will influence the outcome of your labor and the love you have to give to your baby. Unresolved grief over the death of a previous baby or an abortion can prevent your love energy from flowing. Through emotional release, hypnosis, rebirthing, and other counseling techniques, a good therapist can help you to overcome many of these obstacles.

If your ambivalence borders on negativity, this might not be the right time for you to have a baby. If you wait until you feel more enthusiastic, you may be rewarded by a healthier, more enthusiastic child.

There is yet another subtle factor to consider in terms of wanting a baby. Many people do not simply want a baby; they want a baby of a particular sex.

Dr. Thomas Verny did a pilot study about the interrelationship between the mother's attitude about childbearing and the sexual gender of her offspring. He found that the best combination for personality development was a positive pregnancy attitude and getting a child of the desired sex. This produced less depression, less irrational anger, and better sexual adjustment.

I can confirm this from my own work. I have seen a lot of grief and confusion about sex roles and sexually related unhappiness among clients whose mother or father very decidedly wanted a child of the opposite sex.

If you have a strong desire for a child of a particular sex and if you cannot see yourself relating positively to a child of the opposite sex, perhaps you should seek counseling.

SINGLE PARENTING

There are individuals who choose to have a baby even though they don't have a regular partner. Most women want to have a good, stable, loving relationship before they have a child. But if a woman can't find such a relationship, and if she longs to have a child, she may opt to have a baby without having a mate.

It may be easier to choose single parenting than to become unexpectedly single. Given the choice, most kids like to have both parents living with them. But a broad survey taken by Dr. Harold A. Minden, author of *Two Hugs for Survival, Strategies for Effective Parenting*, showed that 32 percent of single-parent families found parenting to be fulfilling and positive. That may not sound like a lot, but only 22 percent of two-parent families found parenting to be fulfilling and positive!

Single parents seem to consider parenting either very good or very bad. Among the two-parent families, 42 percent found parenting frustrating, compared to 46 percent of the single-parent families. In the "moderately fulfilling" category were 37 percent of two-parent families and only 22 percent of single-parent families.

BEING IN GOOD HEALTH AT CONCEPTION

A major factor in the health of a child is the mother's health *at conception*. The father's health is also vitally important. Perspective parents would do well to exercise or do physical work outdoors each day; sleep enough so you don't feel tired when you wake up; don't overeat, avoid refined foods (especially white sugar, white flour, and white rice); avoid junk foods and packaged foods made with chemicals, preservatives, and artificial flavorings; and eliminate coffee, cigarettes, and drugs.

Carrying a baby puts a strain on a woman's calcium supply, so have your teeth checked and try to get your dental work done before you conceive. If there are x-rays to be taken (look for a dentist who takes minimal x-rays), make sure they put a protective apron over your abdomen. Don't have x-rays at all unless they're really necessary.

If you've been using birth control pills, wait at least three months before you try to conceive, because the changing hormone cycles can cause spontaneous abortions. Please see the discussion of herbs, food and drugs, and environmental hazards to avoid during pregnancy in chapter 2. Many of these substances should also be avoided for at least a few months before conception.

Maintaining Health and Fertility
If you are just *thinking* about having a baby at some time in the future, and you are concerned about your age, there are things you can do to prolong your health and fertility.

Natural Birth Control
You should be aware of the possible long-term effects of contraceptives on your fertility. Birth control pills work by blocking the production of ovarian hormones, so that ovulation cannot take place. Some women who have taken the pill for over five to ten years have experienced reduced fertility, some have had no periods whatsoever, and some have been rendered sterile.

The IUD works by irritating the lining of the uterus so the fertilized egg won't implant. When the uterus has been irritated every month for a number of years, it can become difficult to conceive.

Condoms and diaphragms and the Ovulation Method (see index) are noninvasive methods of birth control which will not affect your future fertility.

If you are healthy and don't smoke, drink, or use drugs, and you observe the following regimen, beginning in your thirties, you can hope to maintain the optimum health of your reproductive organs and hence your fertility for far longer than the average woman.

Dong Quai and Fasting

Dong Quai (also spelled Dom Kwai or Tang Kuei; the Latin is *Angelica sinensis* or *Angelica polymorpha*) is primarily a Chinese herb, the female counterpart of ginseng. It contains plant substances that are similar to female hormones and it is used to strengthen and restore the female organs. Dong Quai is not generally recommended for use during pregnancy or for women with excessive menstrual flow. It is popular in China for restoring the female organs after childbirth and for easing the changes of menopause. This is an excellent herb for regulating the periods. It is used for purifying the blood and strengthening the circulation. You can buy the whole dried root at herb stores, including Chinese herb stores.

One of the best ways to take dong quai is in combination with fasting. Ideally, set aside one to two weeks (or at least two or three days), preferably in the spring or autumn, and try to fast or eat a simple diet (just fruits and vegetables, for example). During this time, drink plenty of teas and/or juices, including two or three cups of dong quai tea per day.

> **Dong Quai Tea.** Boil 6 cups of water in a pot. Then add 1 medium-size or large root. If you like, you can also add about 1 tablespoon of licorice root, about ½ inch of cinnamon stick, and 1 tablespoon of fresh grated ginger root. These other herbs are health-giving and they add flavor to the tea. Simmer for at least 20 minutes, replacing the water as it evaporates.

You can begin such a program of fasting and drinking dong quai tea at the age of thirty, once a year, and after thirty-five, twice a year — unless you are in poor health or have smoked more than ten cigarettes a day for over a year or otherwise abused your body, in which case you might do it as frequently as four times a year, until your health is restored.

If you cannot fast, take dong quai occasionally, especially when your periods are irregular or more uncomfortable than usual. Nibble off a pea-size piece of the root once or twice a day (if you prefer, you can prepare tea and drink one or two cups per day). Do this for three to ten days before your period is due. Depending on your health, you may want to do this every month, or just a few months per year.

Another way to maintain your fertility is by strengthening your endocrine glands, as explained under "Difficulty Conceiving."

PREGNANCY AFTER THIRTY

There is definitely a movement among women and men toward delaying childbirth until they are in their thirties, or older. We've all heard of the danger involved; just how serious is this?

Some reports say that older women are having fewer complications than previously. I believe this is because older women are becoming more conscious of their health and are better prepared for pregnancy.

Until recently, women were given a long list of statistics concerning things that could go wrong, which became increasingly discouraging for older women. Now there are researchers who take the emphasis off of the woman's age and place it on her individual medical history (herstory) and her present state of health.

The problem with statistics is that they're given for all women. A healthy woman of thirty-five or forty who eats well, is not overweight, has a strong heart and kidneys and no fibroid tumors stands a very good chance of having a fine pregnancy and birth. However, the four most common diseases of aging (diabetes, kidney problems, heart disease, and high blood pressure) are dangerous during pregnancy unless they are managed correctly, beginning in early pregnancy.

Gail Sforza Brewer and her husband, Dr. Tom Brewer, have successfully minimized complications of pregnancy in women of all ages by a common sense program of high-quality nutrition, preparation for childbirth, and the avoidance of drugs and smoking during pregnancy. They cite a study by Dr. Lawrence R. Wharton that shows that even for women over fifty, general health is more important than age in determining the outcome of a pregnancy. The Brewers' excellent program is described in Gail Brewer's thorough book, *The Pregnancy-After-30 Workbook*, (Rodale Press). Another wonderful resource is *You're Not Too Old to Have a Baby* by Jane Price (Penguin Books).

Possible Physiological Problems of Older Parents

Lower Fertility

Some people are extremely fertile and remain that way for a long time. Others have difficulty conceiving at any age. In most cases, a woman's fertility will drop throughout her forties, and she will enter menopause sometime in her fifties. Male fertility also falls during a man's forties, and after forty a man tends to be less fertile than he was at twenty. After the age of fifty, most men have fewer and less active sperm, less testosterone, and are slower to arousal.

If both partners have reduced fertility, then conception will be more difficult. About 15 percent of all couples in the United States have difficulty conceiving. About 30 to 40 percent of the time, the problem lies with the man. If a man wants to test his fertility, he can go to a urologist. He should not assume that he is fertile just because he was ten years ago.

A woman's fertility is much more difficult to assess. If her periods are irregular or painful, or if she has had repeated PID (pelvic inflammatory disease) or mild endometriosis, she may have lower fertility.

Toxemia

This is a syndrome of edema, high blood pressure, and protein in the urine. The early stage is called preeclampsia, and if it begins early in pregnancy, it can cause malformations; later it can cause low birth weight or death of the baby. The most severe stage, eclampsia, is rarely seen.

Statistics show twice as many cases of toxemia among women bearing their first child (primigravidas) in their late thirties as compared to primigravidas in their twenties. Yet Dr. Tom Brewer has shown that women with excellent nutrition have no preeclampsia, no eclampsia (toxemia), no premature babies, and their babies rarely die.

Fibroids

Fibroids are common benign tumors in the uterus. They are increasingly common after the age of thirty. Consult your physician to determine if you have fibroids, and if so, where they are located and whether they might interfere with pregnancy, labor, or delivery.

Down's Syndrome

Down's syndrome, or mongolism, is a well-known birth defect which is characterized by some, though not necessarily all, of the following: a small, flattened skull; a short, flat-bridged nose; wide-set eyes (it's called mongolism because the foregoing are also characteristics of the Mongolian race); short, broad hands and feet with a wide gap between the first and second toes; a little finger that curves inward; underdeveloped genitals; congenital heart defects; below average height; and some degree of mental retardation.

Statistics are damning for the older couple when it comes to Down's syndrome. Until recently, the mother's age was believed to be the only significant factor in the occurrence of this genetic disease. Women were told that they older they were, the greater their chances were of having a Down's syndrome baby. Statistically, the chances for a mother under twenty are only one in 2,500; for a mother in her twenties, they're about one in 1,500. For the mother aged thirty to thirty-four, her chances are about one in 850, and between thirty-five and thirty-nine they mount to one in 280. Between forty and forty-four, her chances are one in 100, and after forty-five, they're one in 40. For a long time it was believed that only the mother's age affected the occurrence of this birth defect, but then it was found that in about one-quarter of the cases, the extra chromosome that caused the defect came from the father.

A new light is being shed on this phenomenon by a study done in 1984 in Scotland by Campbell and Ogston. The parents of 145 children with Down's syndrome were studied with the intention of finding out which factors contribute to the likelihood of having a Down's child. First, they found that only about one-third of the parents were over thirty-five. Medical records of these parents for the years preceding the births were examined and screened for various contributing factors, such as number of miscarriages, problems with infertility, thyroid disease, and exposure to radiation. None of these were found more frequently among the Down's parents than among the controls.

But they did find that both mothers and fathers of Down's children had significantly more illnesses before conception. The mothers were shown to have taken significantly greater amounts of drugs than the control group, including birth control pills, analgesics, antihistamines, hormones, iron supplements (probably iron salts), vaccines, and antibiotics. The Down's mothers also had more than 50 percent greater incidence of psychosis, neurosis, or suicide attempts before conception. Yet another study indicated that a large proportion of Down's mothers had been under severe stress before conceiving their child.

These studies give new hope to older people who are in good health. While it's true that most older people have more illness, take more drugs, and live under more tension than people in their twenties, if these factors do not apply to you, then your chances of having a child with Down's syndrome are greatly diminished.

TEENAGE MOTHERS

Teenage pregnancies present many potential problems. According to the U.S. Department of Health, Education and Welfare, teenage mothers have higher death rates, more hemorrhage, anemia, toxemia, low birth weight babies, and babies with birth defects than women in their twenties. But if you really want to have a baby and you are mature, in good health, and you have an excellent diet, you can expect to have a good pregnancy. Be sure to attend childbirth classes and give plenty of attention to your health and your baby.

Don't be discouraged by statistics. They're given for all women, and no distinction is made between women who want to have their babies and those who don't. It has been shown that mothers who have a positive attitude toward their pregnancy are more likely to have physically and mentally healthy children. Also, statistics do not account for women who have good diets and those who don't.

In fact, many of the negative statistics for teenage mothers are similar to those for women over thirty. For this reason, one of the best books you can read is *The Pregnancy-Over-30 Workbook*, which tells how to manage your diet and your pregnancy.

Having an excellent diet and refraining from smoking and drinking takes you out of the high-risk category, and gives you an excellent chance of having a pleasant pregnancy, a good birth, and a healthy child.

TESTING FOR BIRTH DEFECTS
AND CONGENITAL PROBLEMS

There are various tests that can be given before conception and during early pregnancy to determine if your child will be healthy. If you have good reason to fear that your child will not be normal, you may want to consider the following tests.

If you find that the fetus has a birth defect or congenital problem, you'll have to make a decision about what to do. Don't let doctors or other people pressure you into having an abortion, unless that's really what you want. Consider the matter carefully. If you are thinking about having an abortion, please read my book, *A Difficult Decision, A Compassionate Book About Abortion* (The Crossing Press).

Genetic Counseling
Genetic diseases can be anticipated by examining your family trees. If there are incidents of such diseases in either family, then you may want to consult a genetic counselor. A March of Dimes office or your local hospital can help you locate such a counselor.

Blood Tests
These can determine for Blacks if they are carriers of sickle cell anemia, or if Ashkenazi Jews are carriers of Tay-Sachs disease.

Amniocentesis
Amniocentesis enables a doctor to penetrate the womb to extract a small amount of amniotic fluid, which is cultured for three to four weeks and then examined microscopically. Since the baby's cells shed freely (as ours do), there are free-floating cells in this fluid. The chromosome structure is repeated in every cell. Various birth defects and abnormalities can be detected by examining the cells. For example, Down's syndrome is caused by an extra chromosome. By testing the chemical composition of the amniotic fluid, it can be determined whether the fetus has certain metabolic disorders and several severe congenital abnormalities, such as spina bifida, can be ruled out. Through a combination of amniotic fluid analysis and ultrasound examination, most open neural tube defects can be diagnosed.

During the last three months of pregnancy, amniocentesis can be used to determine if the baby is being endangered by Rh blood disease, diabetes, or toxemia. If there has been premature rupture of the membranes, they can culture the fluid to determine if there is an infection. They can tell if the baby is getting enough oxygen. And the age of the fetus can also be determined, in case an early delivery is required.

The sex of the infant is also known with amniocentesis, so you'll want to decide beforehand whether you want to be told. Many parents were surprised to find that they regretted being told the sex of their future child — it took away part of the mystery for them.

Amniocentesis is usually performed between the thirteenth and sixteenth weeks, so there will be enough amniotic fluid to make the tap. The abdomen is anesthetized and a thin, hollow needle, four inches long, is passed through the uterus. The test feels similar to a blood test.

This procedure has some disturbing side effects. One to three percent of the women who have amniocentesis will experience a miscarriage at some time after the procedure (some of these miscarriages would have occurred anyway). There is some possibility of puncturing the placenta, the cord, or the baby's body. If it isn't done properly, it may cause infection or bleeding of the mother. A British study by the Medical Research Council on pregnant women who had received amniocentesis showed higher rates of hemorrhage after giving birth and more respiratory distress and major orthopedic deformities in the newborns. And finally, it's expensive.

Ultrasound has minimized some of these potential hazards by enabling the physician to locate the baby's exact position, which should be followed immediately by the tap, because if the mother gets up and walks around, the baby may reposition itself. However, ultrasound is an experimental method which has not necessarily been proven to be safe (See Index).

Once the fluid is extracted (in about one case out of 100, this is not successful), it is sent to a lab. Then it takes two to five weeks to get results.

You've already had to wait thirteen to sixteen weeks for the amniocentesis, so you are well into your second trimester, with a fetus of fifteen to twenty-one weeks (nearly four to five months old). After the twelfth week, the usual vacuum curettage abortion is no longer an option. The walls of the uterus are thinner, softer, and spongier, increasing the risk of perforation and excessive bleeding. Any abortion can be disturbing, but when it happens in the second trimester, it is far more traumatic.

Chorionic Villi Sampling

This new method of prenatal diagnosis is an alternative to amniocentesis. At the time of this writing it is still in the experimental stage. A small sample is taken from the developing placenta (which can be reached by going in through the vagina). These cells are examined in a lab to analyze the fetal chromosomes. Because the embryo and placenta are both formed from cells of the original fertilized egg, this method (combined with a small blood sample and ultrasound) is comparable to amniocentesis (combined with ultrasound). In centers where the physician is experienced, a sample can be obtained in about 96 percent of the cases.

The greatest advantage of CVS is that it can be done early in the pregnancy, so that a woman will have the results and be ready to consider an abortion at ten to fourteen weeks (three to three-and-a-half months), which means that she may still be able to have a vacuum abortion — a procedure which takes about ten minutes when it's performed in a clinic.

Because CVS is so new, there is little information about the safety and accuracy of the test. Based on limited experience in Europe and the United States, three to four out of every one hundred women having CVS may have a miscarriage at some time following the procedure.

DIFFICULTY CONCEIVING

According to Dr. Robert Kolodny, coordinator of the Masters-Johnson Reproductive Biology Research Foundation, one out of every eight couples in the U.S. has difficulty conceiving. In at least forty percent of these cases, the situation is caused either wholly or in part by low sperm production.

If you are having trouble conceiving, consider your health, your habits, and your environment. You and your partner should both see a doctor to determine if you are both in good health. The man should have a sperm count taken.

Read about "Substances for Men to Avoid or Minimize" in chapter 2 and about the herbs, food and drugs, and environmental hazards women should avoid in chapter 2. Many of these substances are known to lower fertility in both men and women. If you have minimized most of these substances for at least one year and you're still having trouble conceiving, there are other things you can do.

When you're quite certain that you want a child, if you're in good health, you will probably get pregnant soon with the following methods. But if you try these methods conscientiously for three months without results, consult a doctor who is a specialist in fertility.

1. Regulate Your Periods and Determine Your Fertile Days

If your periods aren't regular, it's difficult to anticipate your fertile days. So the first step is to try to regulate your periods.

Dong Quai

This Chinese herb is the female equivalent of ginseng, which is well known as the longevity and virility herb for men. Dong quai contains plant substances that are similar to female hormones. It's good for the female organs, though it should not be taken during pregnancy. Dong quai can be purchased at most herb stores, including Chinese herb stores. Usually it is sold as a dried root. Nibble off a pea-sized piece of the root twice a day. Your period will probably become regular within a month or two. Then you will probably need to continue taking the herb for three to ten days before each period is due. But after you stop using birth control, discontinue using this herb.

Lunaception

This is a method of regulating your menstrual cycle. It is based on the observation that the light-sensitive pineal gland, which is located in the central part of the brain, behind the "third eye," plays a role in regulating ovulation. Many years ago Louise Lacey did some research which suggested that before the advent of electricity, women had "moon cycles"; that is, they ovulated and menstruated in relation to the full and the new moon. Ms. Lacey speculated that electricity has thrown off women's menstrual cycles.

I was interested in her theory, because I noticed that women who live in rural areas (away from city lights) often menstruate at the same time, usually at the new or full moon.

Perhaps it is the stimulation of this gland by light which explains why farmers can induce chickens to lay more eggs by putting a light on in the chicken coop at night.

Louise Lacey found a study conducted at the John Rock Reproductive Clinic for infertile women in which women slept with a one-hundred-watt light on the floor at the foot of their beds for the fourteenth, fifteenth, and sixteenth nights of their menstrual cycles, counting the first day of their period as day one. They found that previously irregular, infertile women were able to regulate their ovulation cycles into a regular twenty-nine-day rhythm, ovulating predictably on the fourteenth or fifteenth day. They experimented with using the light on various other nights, but they found that only this formula worked effectively. Ms. Lacey noticed that this rhythm followed the same pattern as the moon cycles, with the light bulb mimicking the nights that the moon was full or nearly full.

Experimenting with herself and eighteen willing friends, Louise Lacey found that they could regulate their monthly menstrual periods. They also found that by using this method, their periods kept perfect rhythm with the new and full moons—except when they were under severe stress. She found that this method could be used effectively both for getting pregnant and for birth control. (But she cautioned that Masters and Johnson found that there were some highly fertile women who sometimes ovulated when they had an orgasm. She said that these women would notice irregularities in their charting, and that this method of birth control would not work for them.)

Here is the method.

1) Prepare Your Bedroom. It is essential to sleep in complete darkness ordinarily. So you may need to buy heavy drapes or a shade, or put a cloth along the crack at the bottom of your bedroom door. Then you will need a low power light source, such as a fifteen-watt night-light, plugged into a socket near your bed, or a forty-watt bulb in the closet, or a dim hall light to use three nights a month. It should not be bright, but it should be perceptible through closed eyelids.

2) Make a Chart. Buy plain quarter-inch-ruled graph paper. Position it so that the long side runs from left to right. On the far left column, leave two blank lines at the bottom and then, moving upward, write a list of temperatures, by tenths, going from 97.5° F., and then on the next line up, 97.6°, and then 97.7°, and up to 100.0° at the top.

Along the top, one to a square, list the dates starting with the date you begin using the chart. You may want to wait until the end of your current menstrual cycle.

3) Take Your Temperature Daily. Buy a good-quality oral thermometer. Don't buy the cheapest, regardless of guarantees, because the temperature needs to be exact, and the cheap thermometers are not reliable. Decide on a time of day when you will take your temperature. The important thing is to do it the same time every day, within about 15 minutes. So if you get up early during the week and you sleep in on the weekends, it might be more reliable to do it around dinner time. Do not smoke, eat, drink, or brush your teeth for ten minutes beforehand. Leave the thermometer in your mouth, under your tongue, for at least four minutes (this may not be relevant with a digital thermometer). If you have a cold or other infection, or if you're under severe stress, your temperature may not be normal. So you need to chart your temperature for at least three months before you can be sure of a pattern. Make a dot on the graph in the column below the date, exactly opposite the temperature the thermometer shows. Draw a line from from one dot to the next.

4) Use the Light. You will need to know what day the moon is full. Many calendars indicate the time of the full moon, or you can get an astrological calendar. Count the day of the full moon as day fifteen, and then on the nights of days fourteen, fifteen, and sixteen, sleep with your light on (if you live in the country where there are no artifical lights, just leave your curtains open). On all other nights, sleep in a darkened room. (If you live in the country, you can still leave your curtains open.) Within a few months, you should be ovulating with the full moon (however, some women mensturate with the full moon and ovulate two weeks later with the new moon).

5) Read the Chart. When ovulation occurs, there is a change in your hormones which will be reflected in your daily temperature. There will be a slight fall, followed the next day by a steep rise by as much as a whole degree or more. This is called a phase shift. The temperature will then stay high, varying as much as a full degree up or down, until the next period, when it will fall back to the original temperature. When your period becomes regulated with the light, the phase shift will occur predictably the night before you sleep with the light on.

While a phase shift covers a period of forty-eight hours, ovulation takes only a few seconds, and the fertility of the egg only lasts for about eight hours. Since you cannot know which eight of the forty-eight are fertile, you should take advantage of the whole period. Also, sperm can live for forty-eight hours inside a woman's body, so if you are using this as birth control, you should abstain from sexual relations or use some other form of contraception for at least a full five days—two days before you use the light (before the anticipated phase shift) and the three days you use it. Do not rely on this as a form of contraception until your cycles are reliably regular. The only really safe way to use this method is to wait until you have definitely ovulated, and then wait another three days after that. Before ovulation you can use another form of birth control.

The Ovulation Method
This is another method for determining your fertile days. It can be used in conjunction with Lunaception, or it can be used separately. It is also used for birth control. The Ovulation Method is based on the knowledge that estrogen increases in a woman's body until it reaches its peak, at which time another hormone, luteinizing hormone, is released, causing an ovum to erupt from the ovary and to begin its journey down the fallopian tube, where it can be fertilized. At this time the rise in estrogen level causes the os (the mouth of the uterus, through which the sperm must travel to reach the ovum) to open up. During this time the ovulation mucus stretches itself into a corridor pattern that leads the sperm directly up to the uterus. These corridors vibrate within the same frequency range as the tails of the sperm! The ovulation mucus is richly supplied with glucose, to nourish the welcomed sperm, so that they may live and fertilize for as long as five and a half days.

Ovulation mucus not only enhances the possibility of conception, it is a prerequisite for it. After ovulation, the tacky, sticky cervical mucus sets in and the os closes up. Then the cervical mucus blocks the cervix and the closed os with a cobweb pattern of mucus which helps prevent the sperm from getting through. This kind of mucus is high in leukocytes (white blood cells) which surround the sperm and ingest them. It also contains anti-trypsin. Trypsin is an enzyme in the head of the sperm which enables the sperm to break down the outer shell of the egg and enter it. Finally, this mucus also contains factors which tend to clump the sperm and stop the movement of their tails. Most sperm cannot survive more than a few hours in such an unfriendly medium.

The challenge, then, is to learn to identify the ovulation mucus. There are two kind of secretions in a healthy woman's vagina: the secretion produced in response to sexual stimulation, and the cervical mucus which comes down from the cervix (the neck of the uterus). Just before ovulation, this cervical mucus resembles egg white; it feels slippery and it can be "stretched" without breaking. To test this, insert your index or third finger slightly into your vagina and get some mucus on your finger, then touch your thumb to the mucus and slowly move your thumb away from your finger. The mucus should stretch out in long strands between the two fingers. You may notice this slippery mucus when you wipe yourself after urinating.

After observing your mucus for a full cycle between periods, you'll become aware of the changes it undergoes. You can learn to identify the ovulation mucus, and then, if your observation is correct, the menstrual period will begin eleven to sixteen days after the ovulation mucus becomes most stretchy. Since semen closely resembles the consistency of ovulation mucus, instructors ask women to abstain for one month before using the ovulation method in order to observe their mucus without confusion.

This method works even if your periods are irregular, or if you are coming off the pill, or if you have just had a baby. By observing the mucus each day, you can tell when you are ovulating. This method should be used in conjunction with the charting described under Lunaception. Each day you can mark on the chart whether your mucus is tacky or slippery.

If you want to use the Ovulation Method for birth control, it is strongly recommended that you find an instructor. Classes usually involve a two-hour presentation with follow-up about a month later. To obtain the names of teachers in your area, send a self-addressed, stamped envelope to The Ovulation Method Teacher's Association, P.O. Box 14511, Portland, Oregon 97214. (See Recommended Books for a list of books on natural birth control.)

2. Strengthen Your Endocrine Glands

Vitamins A and E. These vitamins are necessary for the optimum health of your endocrine glands, which regulate ovulation and influence sexual energy. Both the man and woman should take 10,000 I.U. of vitamin A and 800 units of alpha tocopherols each day. Fish liver oil, which is one of the richest sources of vitamin A, is a time-honored remedy among native people for women who are having difficulty conceiving.

Licorice and Sarsaparilla. A tea made of these herbs will strengthen the woman's endocrine glands. Drink one to two cups per day. Store in the refrigerator. You can drink it cold. It is a pleasantly sweet drink.

> **Licorice and Sarsaparilla Tea.** Boil 6 cups of water and add 2 tablespoons of each herb. Simmer for 20 minutes and then strain.

3. Acupressure

In Chinese medicine, the kidney meridian governs the sexual energy. The end of a meridian is a powerful point. The kidney meridian ends at the center of the ball of the foot; it will be tender at that spot. With your thumb, press firmly at this spot while making a clockwise movement. This (or almost any other form of pressure) can be repeated on each foot for up to three minutes every day. Several women who had trouble getting pregnant conceived within a month after using this pressure point. Don't hesitate to try it; there's no harm done if you get the wrong spot.

4. Effective Positioning

This method usually works for women who know when they ovulate. The idea is to place your uterus in the optimum position to receive the sperm and then give the sperm ample time and the assistance of gravity to reach their destination. This is especially effective when the man has low sperm production or low sperm motility.

For one week before you expect to ovulate, don't have sex, but do flirt. This makes the sperm strong and concentrated and makes the woman more receptive.

On the day of ovulation, do not drink any liquids because you will not be able to urinate for a long time after intercourse. You should be sure to urinate before having intercourse.

Lie on your back with your knees up toward your chest. This facilitates deep penetration and helps to create a pool of sperm around the cervix. After the man ejaculates, he should gently withdraw his penis.

Then try to maintain the same position for as long as possible — more than four hours is best. You can put your feet up against the wall and have your partner pile cushions under your legs and all around you. Arrange to have a good book, TV, and music nearby. It's okay to eat, but avoid salty foods because you don't want to drink. Avoid liquids because you don't want to urinate. If this method sounds quite impossible because you tend to urinate frequently, consider placing a disposable incontinent pad or disposable diaper under you.

Try to repeat this procedure again after twenty-four to thirty hours (but not sooner). And again after forty-eight to sixty hours. It usually works the first month, but don't give up until you've tried for two or three months.

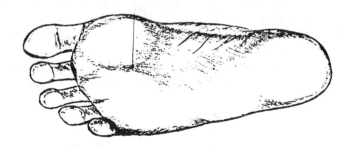

PREGNANCY TESTS

Planned Parenthood offices can be found in most cities. They can tell you which tests are available in your area and where to go to obtain them. Doctors, clinics, and hospitals also offer pregnancy tests. Or you can buy a home test kit from your local drugstore.

HCG Test

This is a laboratory test that checks a woman's urine for the hormone Human Chorionic Gonadotrophin, which is manufactured by the body during pregnancy. You must wait forty-five days after your last menstrual period (forty-five days LMP) to take the test. If your periods are on a regular cycle, that would be about two weeks after your missed period or six weeks from your last actual period. Results are obtained shortly after taking the test.

Home Pregnancy Test

This is a urine test that is available in drugstores. It can be used thirty-nine days after the first day of your last menstrual period, but medical workers say it's possible to get a false negative unless you wait until the forty-fifth day. In some women, the body does not manufacture sufficient HCG to show up on the test until the forty-fifth day. Results are obtained shortly after taking the test.

Early Urine Test

This can be used two weeks after conception, i.e., as soon as your period is missed (four weeks LMP). It takes seven minutes to get the results. This is a relatively new test, so it is not widely available.

Blood Test

This is now available in most large cities. The monoclonol antibody test can be done four to seven days after conception (three weeks LMP). The RIA (radio immuno assay) can be done fourteen days after conception (four weeks LMP) or when the period is one day late. You'll probably need a doctor's referral. These test are more expensive than the early urine test, and when you go to a doctor's office, a result can be obtained in about twenty-four hours. If you go directly to a laboratory, you can have the results from the monoclonal antibody test in about seven minutes. The RIA takes a little longer.

GETTING SETTLED

The nesting instinct is real. Most women like to settle down to have a baby. As a woman enters her last trimester, she will probably want to know where she's going to deliver her baby, and who's going to be there.

During pregnancy, many women change their homes — usually to a larger home, to accommodate the growing family. Yet moving — especially to a whole new location — is a major stress. The mother becomes so preoccupied with setting up her new home that she doesn't have much energy for her child (or her unborn child). If you want to move, do so as early in your pregnancy as possible. If you are six months or more pregnant, be sure to take extra time to pay attention to the baby inside your belly, and get plenty of rest. Remember that the bond that forms between you and your child, both before and after the birth, will influence the relationship you have with that child for the rest of your lives.

Environmental Factors

When people plan to have a family, they become more conscious about the environmental factors that will affect the health of their offspring. There are far more deformed babies being born now than there were twenty-five years ago, and many of these birth defects are environmentally related. So try to locate your home as far as possible from nuclear reactors, uranium mines, chemical dumps, and areas where highly toxic herbicides are commonly used. And when highly polluting industries threaten to move into your neighborhood, remember that someone has to act in behalf of the unborn children.

Staying Home After the Birth

A new mother needs a *minimum* of two weeks to recover from childbirth. In some communities, the neighbors will come in to clean or leave food for the new family, or one of the grandmothers will come and help out for a week or two. If the father is working and can get paternity leave, this can be a great help.

Most newborns don't like being exposed to too many people. They're so open and receptive that they become overstimulated by too much input. Lying quietly in bed with their mother and suckling is their ultimate bliss. Why not give our babies (and ourselves) such simple pleasures? Try to avoid changing homes for *at least* three months before and three months after your baby is born.

REFERENCES

Ernest L. Abel, Ph.D., "Smoking and Pregnancy," *Journal of Psychoactive Drugs*, 16, No. 4, (October-December) 1984.

Gail Sforza Brewer, *The Pregnancy-After-30 Workbook* (Rodale Press, 1978).

Irwin D. J. Bross et al, "Genetic Damage from Diagnostic Radiation," *Journal of the American Medical Association*, 237, No. 22, (May 30) 1977.

Linda Clark, *The Best of Linda Clark* (Keats Publishing, Inc., 1976).

Paul Cressman, "Reproduction Under Siege," *Chimo*, (December) 1981.

Adelle Davis, *Let's Get Well* (Harcourt, Brace and World, 1965).

Joy Gardner, *A Difficult Decision — A Compassionate Book About Abortion* (The Crossing Press, 1986).

Joy Gardner, *Healing Yourself*, 7th revised edition (The Crossing Press, 1986).

Grace Hospital and the University of British Columbia in Vancouver, Information Sheet, "U.B.C. Chorionic Villus Sampling (DVS) and Amniocentesis Randomized Trial" (1986).

Louise Lacey, "Lunaception," *CoEvolution Quarterly*, (Winter Solstice) 1974.

Martindale, *The Extra Pharmacopoeia*, 26th edition, edited by Normal W. Blacow (The Pharmaceutical Press, 1972).

Medical World News, "Amniocentesis Kills 1.5% of Fetuses in British Study," February 19, 1976.

Dr. Harold A. Minden, *Two Hugs for Survival, Strategies for Effective Parenting* (McClelland and Stewart, 1984).

J. Campbell Murdoch and S. A. Ogston, "Characteristics of Parents of Down's Children and Control Children with Respect to Factors Present Before Conception," *Journal of Mental Deficiencies Research*, 28, 1984.

Jane Price, *You're Not Too Old to Have a Baby* (Penguin Books, 1977).

William J. Schull, Ph.D. "Reproductive Problems: Fertility, Teratogenesis, and Mutagenesis," *Archives of Environmental Health*, 39, No. 3, (May/June) 1984.

Susan Stern, "A Guide to Worrying Intelligently About Having a Baby," *CoEvolution Quarterly*, No. 21, (Spring) 1979.

Michael Tierra, C.A., N.D., *The Way of Herbs — Simple Remedies for Health and Healing* (Unity Press, 1980).

Thomas Verney, with John Kelly, *The Secret Life of the Unborn Child* (Collins Publishers, 1981).

Chapter 2
Being Pregnant

We tend to think that a baby in utero is entirely cut off from the world that lies just beyond a thin layer of skin. We seldom consider the child within as a conscious being, capable of responding to sounds, emotions, and the inner environment that its mother creates through her sense of well-being, or lack of it.

In his excellent book, *The Secret Life of the Unborn Child*, Dr. Thomas Verny tells an uncanny story about a man who had a startling recollection while under medication. This man recalled being in an enclosed room. It was a pleasant sensation, until people began crowding around him, pointing their fingers accusingly at him. He felt angry and frightened and helpless.

He could not make sense of his "memory" until he described it to his mother. She told him that when she was pregnant with him, she was in a roomful of people at a party when several of her friends learned that she, an unmarried woman, was pregnant. Though they said nothing, she felt as if they were all staring at her with condemnation.

Dr. Dennis Stott did a series of studies in which he found that no ill effects—physical or emotional—were apparent in the offspring of women who suffered fairly intense but brief stress during pregnancy. Even prolonged threats were not a problem, if they did not directly threaten a woman's emotional security. But personal stress, such as tension with a husband or an in-law, frequently did have an effect upon the unborn child. This was especially disturbing when it tended to be continuous, or unpredictable, liable to erupt at any time, and basically incapable of resolution. Ten of fourteen women in the study who were subjected to these stresses bore children with physical or emotional problems.

Dr. Verny believes that the intensity of a woman's feeling toward her child can lessen the impact her upsets have on the child. When a child feels shielded by her love, that shielding can decrease or neutralize the impact of outside tensions.

One of my clients whose husband died when she was three months pregnant believed that if she allowed herself to grieve as deeply as she longed to, she would have had no energy to give to her developing baby. So she forced herself to delay her grieving until the child was one year old, and then she left the child with a friend for a few days and went off to grieve by herself.

Not everyone can do that, and not everyone should try. For example, I worked with another woman who was three months pregnant, and she felt blocked in her ability to give love to the child within. She had had an abortion one year before and still felt guilty toward the baby she had aborted. I asked if she had grieved over the abortion, and she said no.

I asked if she wanted to grieve now, and she said she was afraid of hurting her baby. She knew she had a lot of unexpressed anger toward the father of the first baby. I explained that she was doing far more harm to the present baby by not expressing her feelings, because that made her feel numb inside, so the baby couldn't feel her positive energy.

I suggested that she put her hands on her belly and visualize a white light around the baby inside so that it could feel her love and protection. Then I encouraged her to talk about her feelings. I suggested that she vent her anger by hitting cushions. She allowed herself to do that, and then she found that she was able to cry for the baby she had lost.

A week later she wrote and said she was happy at last, and was finally feeling excited about the baby she was carrying.

If something traumatic happens to you while you are pregnant, in most cases, it is best to express your feelings and also maintain your connection with the child within. According to Dr. Verny, anger or anxiety in small doses actually hastens the development of rudimentary intellectual connections. The outside intrusion forces the child out of his or her blankness, concentrates the attention, elicits an emotional response, and produces a memory trace.

But when the mother suffers a major loss that causes her to withdraw her love and support from her unborn child for a prolonged period of time, that loss plunges the child into a depression. Babies whose mothers withdrew from them emotionally while they were in the womb are often born withdrawn and apathetic. Life in the womb is bound completely to the mother. Even outside noises are conducted through her. Her very heartbeat sets the rhythm for the unborn child's daily life. When the mother is at peace, her steady heartbeat is like a constantly reassuring lullaby. This has been demonstrated by playing a tape of the human heartbeat in a nursery filled with newborns. Compared to the babies who did not hear this reassuring, familiar sound, the heartbeat babies ate more, weighed more, slept more, breathed better, cried less, and had less sickness.

By the time the fetus is in its sixth month it can hear perfectly and it may literally jump in rhythm to the beat of an orchestra drum. Many women stop going to concerts because their unborn babies make them feel so uncomfortable.

Verny tells a remarkable story about a cello player who found that he knew certain pieces even before he had read the music. When he described this to his mother (also a cello player), she remarked that those were the pieces she had played most frequently while she was pregnant with him.

One of my clients told me that there were certain passages from the Bible that he dearly loved and easily learned by heart. Later his mother told him that those were the passages that she had read aloud, over and over, during her pregnancy with him.

Verny tells about a woman who found her two-year-old daughter sitting on the living room floor chanting to herself, "Breathe in, breathe out, breathe in, breathe out" in exactly the same pattern that her mother had used for her Lamaze exercises all through her pregnancy and delivery—and not at all since.

With my first child, I was in labor for thirty-six hours. The last several hours were filled with painful contractions. I had been trained in the Lamaze method, and I made good use of the pant-and-blow technique which consists of three short pants followed by a long blow. For several days after my son was born, he had a peculiar habit of taking three short pants followed by a long blow!

I met a woman who had been a political activist while she was pregnant. She was involved in organizing political rallies, and she often stayed up all night, drinking lots of coffee. When her son was three years old, he astonished her by saying, "Mommy, when I was inside your tummy, I tried to tell you to stop drinking all that coffee, but you wouldn't pay any attention to me!"

Modern research with plants shows that they like to be spoken to, and they respond well to certain music, and grow more profusely when they're loved and well cared for. If this is true for a plant, it must be doubly true for the growing human baby.

When a baby is inside its mother's belly, how does he or she feel loved? That growing baby can feel her love when she strokes her belly fondly, when she eats sensibly, when she takes a moment to talk and to sing to the baby, when she notices the baby kicking a certain way and wonders if the little one is uncomfortable or scared, and when the father strokes the mother's belly and says nice things to the baby.

LIGHTENING YOUR WORK LOAD

Many of us see ourselves moving through pregnancy and childbirth, strong as a bull, without ever resting or needing special consideration. But bulls don't have babies, and the strength of pregnancy has a quality of its own. This is a time when a woman needs the strength to nurture, to be patient, and to maintain good nonstrenuous daily exercise. We need the self-discipline *not* to overwork. We need to respect the fragile life within us; to sit or lie down when we have the urge. If we begin to respond to our body's needs in pregnancy, it will be much easier to respond to our baby's needs later.

The strength of pregnancy is unique. I've seen several labors which were so long and intense that the men who were there were awe-stricken as their women rode on the powerful waves of their contractions without anesthesia. So don't be impatient when your body demands rest; it may just be building up its resources for later. What could be more important than the new life you carry? Your body is its house, its cradle, and its nourishment. How you care for yourself will affect the body your child will have for the rest of its life!

EXERCISE

Keeping your body healthy by exercising is vital during pregnancy. Studies show that labor may be shorter for women who are physically fit. But exercise should never be harsh or carried to the point of physical exhaustion. Getting outdoors as much as possible, walking in pleasant surrounds, and swimming are all excellent. Be sure to wear loose, comfortable clothing that allows for free movement.

Your energy may take a nose dive during the first three months (the first trimester) of your pregnancy. By the fourth month, your blood volume and hemoglobin count will go up (during pregnancy your blood supply increases from 25 to 50 percent above the amount you had before you were pregnant) and you'll probably feel a normal amount of energy.

You'll find that your ability to swim is about the same as usual when you are pregnant, but weight-dependent exercises, such as walking and jogging, will require greater effort because of weight gain and an altered center of gravity.

Former athletes experience shorter labor and have lowered rates of threatened abortion, premature labor, and cesarean section than other women. But athletes who maintain high levels of athletic training during pregnancy do experience more complications. Athletes find that after childbearing, their athletic performance is actually improved. However, high levels of work or athletic training should not be attempted while you are nursing, because this produces large amounts of lactic acid which may influence the quality of your breast milk.

Most yoga positions are good for keeping limber. *Prenatal Yoga and Natural Birth* by Jeannine Parvatti describes yoga postures that are appropriate to use during pregnancy.

Kegel Exercises

Kegel exercises are a vital tool to facilitate an easy delivery without tearing and a speedy recovery after birth. They help your vagina and cervix return to their normal size. In fact, some women who practice Kegels regularly require a smaller size diaphragm after giving birth.

The Kegel muscle holds your insides in place, from the tail bone to the pubic bone. It has spincter openings to the bladder, the vagina, and the rectum. When you have good control over this muscle, you can consciously use your vagina to relax, hold hack, or push in order to facilitate labor and prevent tearing. These exercises are helpful to prevent or get rid of hemorrhoids during and after pregnancy. A strong Kegel muscle will also increase your own and your partner's sexual pleasure by facilitating stronger and more pleasurable spasms of orgasm, and because of the pleasant squeezing sensation.

To strengthen your Kegel muscles, try the following exercises:

1. When urinating, just release a small amount of urine and then stop the flow. Repeat several times.
2. Repeat the same hold-release movement several times a day, very slowly, in series of five.
3. Practice contracting the muscle slowly to the count of five.

NUTRITION AND WEIGHT GAIN

A healthy, nutritious diet, with food in moderation or several small meals per day — combined with fresh air, exercise, and a cheerful spirit — almost never fails to turn out beautiful, alert children. But many pregnant women diet severely to prevent weight gain, or eat mostly junk food (this is one reason why teenage mothers often give birth to premature babies), or suffer from malnutrition. This does irreparable damage to their unborn children. I've seen many people who were mysteriously unhealthy despite excellent diets; their ill health could be traced back to their mother's inadequate diet during pregnancy.

The American College of Obstetrics and Gynecology has stated that "the future health of mankind depends, to a very large degree, on nutritional foundations laid down during prenatal life."

How much weight should you gain, and what kinds of foods should you eat? It is now believed that a weight gain of thirty to thirty-five pounds is healthy during pregnancy. In fact, one study showed that women who gained thirty-six pounds or more during pregnancy had the lowest incidence of low birth weight and brain-damaged children.

The amount of weight gained is far less important than the kind of food you eat. If you eat plenty of fresh fruits and vegetables, whole grains, some source of fat (such as cold-pressed unhydrogenated vegetable oil), adequate protein, and if you avoid white sugar, refined foods, deep-fat fried and other junk foods, you can eat according to your appetite.

If you get plenty of exercise, then your weight gain will probably be appropriate to you. The main thing to watch out for is a rapid gain of three to seven pounds in one week, together with edema. This could indicate toxemia. But such a gain would not be caused just by a high intake of calories.

Now — while you are pregnant — is the optimum time to establish good eating habits. The average person in the United States consumes 600 calories of white sugar per day. That's about one-quarter of their daily caloric intake. These are called empty calories because white sugar has no nutritional value.

Refined foods are a poor way to build your baby's body. A large intake of white refined sugar or flour causes your blood sugar to rise so rapidly that your liver and pancreas don't have enough time to convert the carbohydrates to glucose. This causes nervous tension, stress, exhaustion, and a craving for more sugar in order to get another "fix." The more complex carbohydrates such as unprocessed grains, fruits, and vegetables require a longer time for digestion and breakdown to glucose, so the liver and pancreas have enough time to adjust blood sugar levels back to normal.

Excessive sugar interferes with the absorption of calcium and with bone formation. Large amounts of white sugar and white flour cause the brain to manufacture excessive amounts of serotonin, which causes aggressive behavior. Sugar retards the growth of valuable intestinal bacteria, and pregnancy is a time when the intestines are already crowded and need all the help they can get. Sugar increases the need for vitamin B6, which is a vital nutrient during pregnancy. It also interferes with the absorption of protein.

White sugar requires vitamins B and C for its own assimilation. Since white sugar contains no vitamins, it will rob the body of these valuable nutrients. You will be establishing good eating habits for yourself and your family if you can eliminate refined foods from your diet, and if you can minimize your use of other sweeteners, such as honey, maple syrup, molasses, and brown sugar. These contain some valuable vitamins and minerals, but they are fattening and bad for your teeth.

Many midwives have observed that when women eliminate empty calories and junk food from their diet, whatever weight they gain tends to come off fairly easily while they're nursing and after the baby is weaned. But women who gain weight from eating empty foods find that it is difficult to lose the weight they put on during pregnancy.

If you're not satisfied with the food you eat, consider taking a cooking class. Good cooking is an essential part of good nutrition. *Nourishing Your Unborn Child* by Phyllis S. Williams, R.N., combines nutritional information with recipes. *Laurel's Kitchen* by Laurel Robertson is an excellent book on vegetarian cooking and nutrition, and it gives careful instruction on how to change your diet, and why.

As your baby grows larger, you probably won't have enough space for three big meals a day, so be prepared to shift your eating pattern to four or five smaller, balanced meals. Or eat moderately at mealtime, and then concentrate on getting nutritious snacks.

IMPORTANT NUTRIENTS

Vitamin A
This nutrient is necessary for growth, vitality, and proper development and upkeep of the eyes and skin. Lack of vitamin A has been connected with birth

defects. The RDA before pregnancy is 4,000 I.U. During pregnancy it goes up to 5,000, and while nursing it increases to 6,000. If you live in a large city, you may need more because of exposure to pollutants. In the country, exposure to pesticides may increase your need for vitamin A. This vitamin is stored in your liver, so if you get a lot of it one day, you can get by with much less for the next two or three days.

Vitamin A occurs in nonanimal foods in the form of carotene (provitamin A). In order for carotene to be absorbed, food must be chewed very thoroughly. Exposure to air destroys carotene, so juices and grated vegetables should be freshly prepared. In order to get maximum absorption of vitamin A and carotene, it helps to take vitamin E at the same time, to protect the vitamin A from being destroyed by oxygen. Vitamin D, protein, and choline (a B vitamin) also increase the effectiveness of vitamin A. Vitamin A supplements should always be taken with a meal or with milk or some form of fat, because fats stimulate the flow of bile and digestive enzymes, which are essential for the absorption of this vitamin.

The following foods contain about 3,000 I.U. of vitamin A:

Apricots (3 medium-size)
Cantaloupe (½ medium-size)
Mango (½)
Papaya (¼ medium-size)
Persimmon (1 medium-size)
Beet greens (¼ cup cooked or ¾ cup raw)
Chard (¼ cup raw or cooked)
Collards (⅓ cup raw or cooked)
Garden cress (⅓ cup cooked or ⅔ cup raw)
Dandelion greens (½ cup cooked or ⅓ cup raw)
Dock or sheep sorrel (½ cup cooked or ⅓ cup raw)
Kale (½ cup cooked or ⅓ cup raw)
Mustard (¼ cup raw or cooked)
Bok choy cabbage (⅔ cup cooked or 1 cup raw)
Spinach (⅓ cup cooked or ½ cup raw)
Parsley (¼ cup raw)
Pumpkin (½ cup canned)
Winter squash (¼ cup cooked)
Vegetable juice cocktail (⅓ cup canned)
Beef liver (½ ounce)
Calf liver (⅓ ounce)
Pork liver (⅔ ounce)
Liverwurst sausage (1¼ ounces)

Vitamin A supplements are made from fish liver oils and are available in drugstores and health food stores.

Vitamin B

The twelve different substances that compose the B complex form the basis for all cellular growth and multiplication. Lack of B vitamins can cause nervousness, weakness, depression, constipation, anemia, vaginal infections, inability to urinate, and lack of appetite to the point of weight loss. Whenever you're under stress, remember to take extra Bs.

The foods that are highest in B vitamins include brewer's or torula or nutritional yeast, wheat germ, rice polish or bran, blackstrap molasses, and liver. Since it is water-soluble, the vitamin will leach out into the cooking water, so avoid boiling vegetables in water and then throwing out the water. It is better to steam your vegetables. White sugar should be avoided because it uses the body's stores of vitamin B for its own assimilation. Alcohol also destroys B vitamins.

Vitamin B supplements should always be taken as a whole complex instead of taking any B vitamin factor by itself, because the Bs work together, as a team. If you get an excess of one B vitamin, it can throw the others off balance.

Vitamin B complex is commonly obtained in the form of brewer's or torula or nutritional yeast. During pregnancy, find a form of yeast that contains plenty of folic acid. If you're a strict vegetarian, it should also have ample vitamin B12.

Folic Acid. The need for folic acid doubles during pregnancy, from .4 mg. (400 mcg.) to .8 mg. (800 mcg.). A deficiency can lead to toxemia, premature birth, premature separation of the placenta, afterbirth hemorrhaging, and megaloblastic anemia (sore mouth, sore tongue, and sometimes a grayish-brown skin pigmentation known as pregnancy mask) in both mother and child, as well as infant birth defects.

The following foods contain about .1 mg. (100 mcg.) of folic acid:

Fresh orange juice (¾ cup)
Spinach (3 ounces)
Romaine lettuce (1 cup, cut)
Brussel sprouts (3 large)
Broccoli (1 large stalk)
Soy flour (⅓ cup)
Soybeans (¼ cup dry)
Lima beans (½ cup dry)
White kidney beans (⅓ cup dry)
Garbanzo beans (⅓ cup dry)
Brewer's yeast (1 heaping tablespoon)

Liver, kidneys, and chicken giblets are rich sources of this nutrient.

Folic acid is destroyed when you overcook food. When you cook in water, folic acid goes into the water — so don't throw away the cooking water.

Use it for soups or for cooking grains or beans. Long storage of food also destroys this valuable nutrient.

Notice that each of the foods that are high in folic acid provide only one-eighth of your total daily requirement. For this reason, supplementation may be desirable. Try to find a good B complex tablet or a form of yeast that contains at least .8 mg. (800 mcg.) of folic acid. Vitamin C is necessary to enable the body to absorb folic acid.

Vitamin B6 (Pyridoxine). During pregnancy and lactation, your need for this B vitamin increases from 2 mg. to 2.6 mg. per day. Most pregnant women are deficient in B6, which accounts for the following symptoms (which characterize far too many pregnancies): nausea and vomiting (morning sickness), leg cramps, nervousness, lack of energy, insomnia, bad-smelling gas, irritability, hemorrhoids, and anemia.

The following foods contain about .5 mgs. of B6:

Avocado (½ large)
Banana (1 small)
Watermelon (3-inch by 8-inch piece)
Prunes, cooked (⅓ cup)
Beans, including lima, lentils, and soybeans (½ cup cooked)
Mung bean sprouts (1 cup cooked)
Broccoli or Brussel sprouts (2 cups cooked)
Corn (1¼ cups)
Collard leaves (1½ cups steamed)
Peas (¼ cup cooked)
Full-fat soy flour (⅔ cup)
Whole wheat flour (½ cup)
Brown rice (½ cup)
Wheat bran (¼ cup)
Peanuts (⅔ cup)
Beef or pork (4 ounces)
Liver (2⅓ ounces)
Chicken (2⅔ ounces broiled)

Notice that each of the above foods provide only one-fifth of your total daily requirement of B6. This is a strong argument in favor of supplementation, especially before conception and during pregnancy (to prevent or cure morning sickness) and lactation.

While nursing, it may be best to use yeast or B complex pills that contain a smaller amount of B6, because pyridoxine can inhibit the secretion of breast milk by suppressing prolactin production. During lactation, your B6 requirement drops from 2.6 during pregnancy to 2.5. All the other vitamins increase or remain the same during lactation.

Vitamin C

The RDA for vitamin C is 60 mg. for nonpregnant women, 80 mg. while pregnant, and 100 mg. while nursing. However, pregnancy is a stress on the body, and during times of stress the body consumes large amounts of vitamin C. Most pregnant women feel better when they take 500 to 1,000 mg. per day. Any infection, cold, or increased stress is a good reason to temporarily raise the dosage to 1,000 to 3,000 mg. per day. During lactation, it is good to take an additional 500 mg. per day. *Note*: Doses of over 4,000 mg. per day are not recommended during the first three months of pregnancy.

The following foods contain about 50 mg. of vitamin C:

Oranges (½ large)
Tangerines (2½ medium-size)
Grapefruit (½ medium-size fresh or ¾ cup canned)
Grapefruit juice (4 ounces)
Lemons (1 medium-size)
Limes (1½ medium-size)
Papaya (¼ medium-size)
Persimmon (½ medium-size)
Guava (⅓ medium-size)
Strawberries (⅔ cup)
Gooseberries (1 cup)
Loganberries, blackberries, and red raspberries (1⅓ cups)
Black raspberries (1½ cups)
Broccoli (2/5 cup raw or ⅔ cup cooked)
Brussel sprouts (½ cup raw or ⅔ cup cooked)
Cabbage (¼ small head raw or ⅔ cup cooked)
Cauliflower (½ cup raw or ⅔ cup cooked)
Collards (½ cup raw or cooked)
Cress (1½ cups raw or 1⅓ cups cooked)
Dandelion greens (1⅓ cups raw or 1¼ cups cooked)
Dock (½ cup raw or ⅔ cup cooked)
Kale (¼ cup raw or cooked)
Kohlrabi (½ cup cooked or ¾ cup raw)
Lamb's quarters (1 cup raw or cooked)
Mustard greens (¾ cup cooked or ⅔ cup raw)
Okra (1¼ cups cooked or 1 cup cooked)
Parsley (⅓ cup raw)
Hot red chili pepper (½ small raw)
Sweet green pepper (½ medium-size raw)
Rutabagas (⅔ cup cooked or 1 cup raw)
Spinach (1¼ cups raw or cooked)
Tomatoes (2 small, raw or cooked)
Turnips (3 small)
Lima beans and soybeans (1 cup cooked)

We tend to think of citrus as the highest source of this vitamin, and yet papayas, guavas, green peppers, broccoli, and kale are the richest sources of vitamin C.

When this vitamin occurs in nature, it's often in combination with the bioflavanoids (vitamin P). This substance increases the strength of capillaries and regulates their permeability. It helps build healthy collagen (intercellular cement), and it helps prevent hemorrhaging in the capillaries and connective tissues. Therefore it's a very important substance for the mother and the baby, both of whose cells and blood vessels are undergoing constant transformation and growth.

Various brands of Acerola are available in health food stores. These are chewable vitamin C tablets with bioflavanoids. However, when large doses of vitamin C are desired, this can become expensive, so I prefer to take ascorbic acid crystals, a powdered form of ascorbic acid. Usually one-fourth teaspoon contains 1,000 mg. of vitamin C. It's usually sold in large bottles, so the price is fairly high, but it lasts a long time. Ascorbic acid tablets can be purchased at drugstores at a reasonable price. When taking large amounts of ascorbic acid, eat a fresh orange, rose hips, green pepper, or another natural source of bioflavanoids.

Vitamin D

This is necessary for calcium utilization and bone formation. Ordinarily a woman needs 5 mcg. of this vitamin, but during pregnancy and lactation her requirement doubles to 10 mcg. If you are deficient in this vitamin, your child may develop the bowed legs of rickets, resulting in poor growth, bone deformities, poor teeth, and loss of muscle tone. If you live in an area that doesn't get much sun (like the Northwest, in the winter), and if you don't drink vitamin-fortified milk, then be sure to supplement your diet with vitamin D. Vitamin A and D capsules are available at any drugstore at a reasonable price; they're made from fish liver oil, which is a concentrated natural source of vitamins A and D. Other sources of vitamin D are egg yolks, sprouted seeds, mushrooms, and cashew nuts. Sitting in the sun or under a sun lamp every day is another way to get this vitamin, but the ultraviolet light has to mix with the ergosterol (an oily substance) on the skin in order to transform it into vitamin D, which then is absorbed through the skin and goes into the bloodstream. If you bathe, even in cold water, before or after sitting in the sun, this will wash away the ergosterol and prevent the absorption of vitamin D.

Vitamin E, Alpha Tocopherols

This vitamin is essential during pregnancy. The estimated average daily intake of vitamin E is about 14 mg. of alpha tocopherols. The normal RDA is 8 mg., while the RDA during pregnancy is 10 mg., and during lactation, it's 11 mg. If you eat whole grain, unrefined foods, you are probably getting enough vitamin E. But if you have a tendency toward miscarriage, take a supplement of 400 I.U. per day. It's important to use alpha tocopherols, because the mixed tocopherols have not proven as effective in preventing miscarriage.

During labor, if the baby is in the birth canal for a long time, there's a danger of asphyxiation, which is why forceps are often used when labor is prolonged. Vitamin E reduces the oxygen requirement by making maximum use of existing oxygen, so during the last two weeks of pregnancy, take 400 I.U. per day, preventatively.

Vitamin F
This is a term for essential fatty acids which are found in vegetable oils. Little attention is given to fats and oils, yet they're essential for human growth and for the absorption of calcium. One to two tablespoons of vegetable oil per day, raw or cooked, is advisable.

Vitamin K
The RDA for this vitamin does not change during pregnancy and lactation. But vitamin K is essential for proper blood coagulation. Deficiencies can cause miscarriage and lead to hemorrhaging after childbirth. The absorption of vitamin K is hindered by the use of rancid fats, mineral oil, aspirin, oral antibiotics, x-rays, radiation, and chemical vapors. If you're exposed to these things, then the additional intake of vitamin K is advisable.

Alfalfa is an excellent source of this vitamin. However, alfalfa tea does not contain vitamin K because the vitamin does not disperse in water, since it's oil soluble. Alfalfa pills are sold in health food stores.

I suggest taking two to six tablets per day during the last two weeks of pregnancy, to help prevent hemorrhaging. This is especially important if you're a redhead, because redheads have a greater tendency to hemorrhage. Vitamin K is found in all dark green leafy vegetables (kale, cabbage, spinach, nettle, etc.), and tomatoes (especially green tomatoes). The bacteria in the human gut synthesize this vitamin.

Calcium
The RDA for an adult woman is 800 mg. of calcium, but while pregnant and nursing, it jumps to 1,200. If a pregnant mother doesn't get enough calcium, her bones will demineralize; the calcium in her bones will break down and pass into her blood to nourish the baby. This can cause osteoporosis (thinning out of the bones as a woman grows older, resulting in fractures that are very difficult to mend). If calcium is deficient, you may have problems with headaches, nervousness, insomnia, leg cramps, spasms, and greater susceptibility to pain. If the fetus doesn't get enough calcium, your child may have bowed legs, faulty bone structure, and unhealthy, crooked teeth.

The following foods contain about 300 mg. of calcium:

Almonds (1 cup)
Sesame seeds (¼ cup)
Blue cheese (3½ ounces)
Swiss, cheddar, and brick cheese (2 ounces)
Parmesan, American processed, and Swiss processed cheese (1½
    ounces)
Milk (8 ounces)
Greens, including collards, kale, lamb's quarters, dandelion and
    turnip greens (1 to 1½ cups cooked)
Kelp and Irish moss (3 tablespoons)
Tofu or soybean curd (2 cakes)
Second extraction molasses (3½ ounces)
Blackstrap molasses (1½ ounces)
Canned fish with liquids including mackerel (5 ounces)
Sardines and smelt (3 ounces)

Different varieties of salmon have different levels of calcium. To get 300 mg. of calcium, you would have to eat the following amounts of canned or fresh salmon:

Sockeye (3½ ounces)
Chum and Coho (4½ ounces)
Pink (5½ ounces)
Chinook (7 ounces)

Iron

Women need about 18 mg. of iron per day, whether they are pregnant, nursing, or not. During pregnancy, about one-third of your iron supply is taken by the baby to form its blood. Meanwhile, your own blood supply will increase by 25 to 50 percent over the amount you had before pregnancy. This shouldn't cause any trouble, but be sure to have your iron count checked, especially if you're a vegetarian, or if you've had anemia or heavy menstrual flow before pregnancy, or any kind of bleeding during pregnancy.

The iron count is taken by pricking the finger to take blood for a hematocrit, a blood test which indicates the number of red cells in the blood. Red cells carry iron, so a low count may be a sign of iron deficiency anemia. The red cells are also vital because they carry oxygen to your baby's body and your own.

If your hematocrit is below normal, this may indicate a need for more iron, but it may also be caused by a lack of other nutrients that aid in the absorption of iron, such as vitamins B6, B12, folic acid, vitamin C, and magnesium. A more complete analysis of the blood may be advisable if your hematocrit is low. Also, you'll need more than 18 mg. of iron per day to build up your red blood cell count if it is below normal.

Iron salts are discouraged. They interfere with the absorption of vitamin E in the intestines, and since this vitamin is an important oxidizer, the iron salts cut down on your baby's oxygen supply, which can result in miscarriage or premature or delayed birth, or other damage to your baby. Iron salts and vitamin E should not be taken at the same time. If iron salts must be taken, take them at night or in the morning, and take at least 100 I.U. of vitamin E. Allow twelve hours for the vitamin E to be absorbed in your intestines before taking the iron salts. Try to avoid ferrous sulfate and ferrous chloride, which are very harsh on the body. Ferrous fumarate and ferrous gluconate are preferable.

Desiccated liver tablets are a natural source of iron. Most health food stores now carry iron supplements made from entirely natural, organic, non-meat food sources. But, your best source of iron is food. The following foods contain about 5 mg. of iron:

Almonds (¾ cup)
Peanuts (1 cup)
Dry pumpkin and squash seeds (¼ cup)
Dry sunflower seeds (⅔ cup)
Sesame seeds (¼ cup)
Walnuts (1 cup)
Dried apricots (⅔ cup)
Dried peaches (½ cup)
Prunes (1 cup)
Raisins (1 cup)
Beans, including white, red, lima, black-eyed peas, lentils, and
    soybeans (1 cup cooked)
Braised kidney (1 ounce)
Beef liver (2 ounces)
Calf liver (1 ounce)
Pork liver (½ ounce)
Clams (3 ounces)
Oysters (5 medium-size or ⅓ cup)
Tofu or soybean curd (2 cakes)
Greens, including beet greens, chard, dandelion greens, purslane
    leaves, and spinach (1½ cups cooked)
Full-fat soy flour (½ cup)
Molasses, second extraction (5 tablespoons)
Molasses, blackstrap (2 tablespoons)

Protein

It's important to get enough protein, but research now indicates that people in developed countries often get *too much* protein.

Studies of many cultures show that children and adults grow strong and healthy on diets based on single or combined starches. The pictures one sees of "protein-deficient" children are actually pictures of starvation or calorie deficiency. When these children are nursed back to health, it is usually with traditional diets of corn, wheat, rice and/or beans.

The recommendation from the World Health Organization (WHO) for a minimum daily requirement of protein is calculated as approximately 5 percent of your daily calorie intake. During pregnancy, it is 6 percent, and during lactation, it is 6.7 percent. So while a woman is pregnant, she requires an average of thirty-six grams of protein per day, though women who are very active or underweight or pregnant with twins will need closer to forty-five grams. During lactation, the average woman requires an additional two hundred calories, which brings her protein requirement up to forty-three grams. (You can calculate this for yourself by adding the number of calories you consume per day, multiply this by the correct percentage, and divide that by four, since each gram of protein is equal to four calories.)

The WHO recommendation is in sharp contrast to the National Research Council and many reputable nutritionists who recommend seventy-four to one hundred grams of protein per day for pregnant women.

When your diet contains more protein than necessary, it can actually damage your health. The excess protein is broken down in the liver and excreted through the kidneys as urea. Urea has a diuretic effect, causing the kidneys to work harder and excrete more water. When you urinate more frequently than usual, you eliminate important minerals as well as water. One of these minerals is calcium, and calcium is essential during pregnancy and lactation.

Studies of young men on diets of more than ninety-five grams of protein daily showed a negative calcium balance, even when their daily intake of calcium was very high. Studies of adults consuming seventy-five grams of protein a day and as much as 1,400 mg. of calcium per day (far more than the Recommended Dietary Allowance of 800 mg. of calcium per day) showed a negative calcium balance. This helps to explain why 25 percent of women in affluent societies suffer from osteoporosis after the age of sixty-five.

Studies of various cultures show that the higher the protein intake, the more common the occurrence of osteoporosis. Bantus living in Africa on low-protein vegetable diets, consuming forty-seven grams of protein and 400 mg. of calcium, are virtually free of this disease. Native Eskimos who consume 250 to 400 grams of animal protein a day, and over 2,000 mg. of calcium, have one of the highest rates of osteoporosis in the world.

Try to regulate your diet so that you will get enough—but not too much—protein. There are plenty of nonmeat foods that contain about 10 mg. of protein:

LEGUMES

Mung beans (⅓ cup)
Black, garbanzo, pinto or soybeans (½ cup)
Red, white, great northern, lentil, lima, or navy beans, and black-
    eyed or split peas (¾ cup)
Green peas (1¼ cups cooked
Edible pod peas (2 cups)
Soya protein powder (¼ cup) Tofu (4 ounces)

GRAINS AND FLOURS

Soy flour or soy grits (⅓ cup)
Almond meal (½ cup)
Bulgur wheat (¾ cup cooked)
Cracked wheat (1 cup cooked)
Oatmeal (2 cups cooked)
Macaroni (2 cups cooked)
Enriched egg noodles (2 cups cooked)
Dark rye or high protein or soy bread (2 slices)
Date muffins (2)
Corn bread (2 squares)
Pancakes (2)

NUTS AND SEEDS

Pumpkin or squash seeds (¼ cup)
Sunflower seed kernels (¼ cup)
Pine nuts (1 ounce)
Peanuts, cashews, or chopped walnuts (⅓ cup)
Almond or sunflower seed meal (½ cup)
Sesame seed meal (⅔ cup)
Peanut butter (2½ tablespoons)

VEGETABLES

Broccoli (2 medium-size stalks, cooked)
Potatoes (2 medium-size, with skins)
2 cups mashed sweet potatoes or yams (2 cups mashed)
2 medium-size avocados (2 medium-size)
Collard greens, lamb's quarters, or pigweed (1½ cups raw or
    cooked)

DAIRY

Whole cow's milk, skim milk, buttermilk, yogurt, or goat's milk
(1¼ cups)
Low-fat cow's milk or kefir (1 cup)
Dried cow's milk (¼ cup)
Ice cream (1½ cups)
Chocolate malted milk shake (10 ounces)
Ovaltine made with milk (8 ounces)
Cottage cheese, ricotta, or Swiss cheese (⅓ cup)
Cheddar, Edam, limburger, or mozzarella (1½ ounces)
Blue, Roquefort, brick, or Camembert (2 ounces)

MISCELLANEOUS

Eggs (1½ large ones, 6.5 grams each)
Soya protein powder (¼ cup)
Tofu (4 ounces)
Nutritional, brewer's, or torula yeast (3 tablespoons)
Peanut butter (2½ tablespoons)
Bitter or baking chocolate (3 ounces)

Those who eat meat will have no problem consuming enough protein. You
may want to think more about how to limit your protein intake.

MEAT

Dried or chipped beef, kidney, calf liver, lamb liver, or pork liver
(1 ounce)
Hamburger, chuck, lean steak, chicken, turkey, heart, beef liver
(1¼ ounces)
Sirloin steak, corned beef, lamb, veal, tongue (1½ ounces)
Roast beef, duck, pork, ham (2 ounces)
Chili con carne without beans (⅓ cup)
Chili con carne with beans (½ cup)
Stew with vegetables (⅔ cup)

FISH

1 ounce halibut (1 ounce)
Cod, flounder, or canned tuna, drained (1¼ ounces)
Shad, shrimp, or canned salmon, sardines, or mackerel (1½
ounces)
Crab, haddock, scallops (2 ounces)

Clams (2½ ounces)
Kippered herring (½ small)
Lobster (¼ average-size)
Oysters (8 to 10 medium-size or ½ cup)
Oyster stew with milk (1 cup)
Swordfish (⅓ steak)

NUTRITIOUS SNACKS

Getting enough of the proper foods may become difficult as your baby grows and presses on your stomach, limiting its capacity. Nutritious snacks help insure good food intake. Some high-protein snacks are nuts, cottage cheese, cheese slices, yogurt, kefir, and whole grain bread or crackers with unhydrogenated peanut butter and raw honey (a whole protein combination, which is even more nutritious with milk).

The following foods are satisfying, energizing, and excellent sources of iron, calcium, magnesium, protein, B vitamins, and vitamin C.

Tigress Smoothie. You can make a lot at once, store in the refrigerator, and then drink it for a couple days.

¼ to ½ cup whole milk
¼ cup yogurt
Juice of 1 orange (including pulp) or ¼ cup frozen orange juice
    concentrate
1 to 2 tablespoons nutritional yeast
1 to 3 teaspoons molasses
1 tablespoon raw wheat germ
¼ teaspoon vanilla extract
Dash nutmeg

Combine in a blender and process until smooth.

Yogurt Delight. This recipe uses molasses, which is high in nutrients, including iron and calcium, but it's also high in calories.

1 cup of plain yogurt
1 to 2 tablespoons nutritional yeast
1 tablespoon raw wheat germ
1 to 3 teaspoons molasses
Fresh or dried fruit (raisins, apricots, strawberries, bananas, etc.)
2 to 3 teaspoons frozen orange juice concentrate

Spoon the yogurt into a bowl and add the yeast, wheat germ, molasses, and fruit. Top with the juice concentrate, stir, and eat.

HERBS FOR PREGNANCY AND CHILDBIRTH

Throughout history women have used herbs to aid in childbirth. These ancient healing plants are a powerful part of our heritage from the earth. Herbs offer us an opportunity to heal our bodies harmoniously, and they help prepare our bodies in subtle ways for the process of childbirth.

Pregnancy Tea

Raspberry leaf tea is a universal remedy for easing childbirth. This tea is used by pregnant women in North America, South America, Europe, and China. Even pregnant cats will stop to nibble raspberry leaves. Pregnant women were drinking this tea long before scientists discovered that it contains a principle called fragine, which relaxes the smooth muscle of the uterus, making delivery easier and speedier.

The recommended amount depends on when you begin to use this tea. If you begin in early pregnancy, you can take one cup of tea per day throughout your pregnancy. If you begin in the second trimester, you'll need two cups per day for the remainder of your pregnancy. If you don't begin until your last trimester, you'll want to drink three cups per day.

Pregnancy Tea. To prepare the tea, pour 1 cup of boiling water over 1 teaspoon raspberry leaves. Add 1 teaspoon peppermint or any other tea you like for flavor. Let it steep in a covered pot for 5 minutes. Then strain and drink. Add honey if desired.

In the summer, you may want to freeze the sweetened tea in small ice cube trays and then suck on the ice cubes. When used during labor, these raspberry leaf popsicles will help to keep your mouth from getting dry.

Late Pregnancy Tea

During the last two weeks of pregnancy, many midwives suggest a tea of blue cohosh, squaw vine, raspberry leaf, and peppermint to facilitate delivery. Some herbalists recommend these herbs during the last three months of pregnancy, but I prefer to use them only during the last two weeks, unless an early delivery is desired. If there is any suspicion that the baby may be undersized, this tea should not be used, because you want to be sure that the baby will have the maximum time it needs to grow. This is an excellent tea to use during childbirth. Blue cohosh helps to open the uterine os. Late Pregnancy Tea relaxes the pelvis, which helps ease delivery and lessens the chances of tearing.

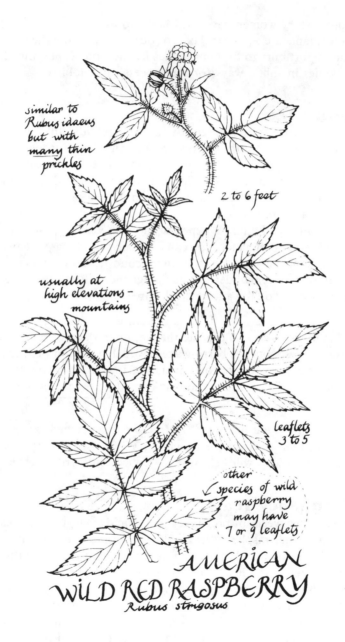

similar to
Rubus idaeus
but with
many thin
prickles

2 to 6 feet

usually at
high elevations —
mountains

leaflets
3 to 5

other
species of wild
raspberry
may have
7 or 9 leaflets

AMERICAN
WILD RED RASPBERRY
Rubus strigosus

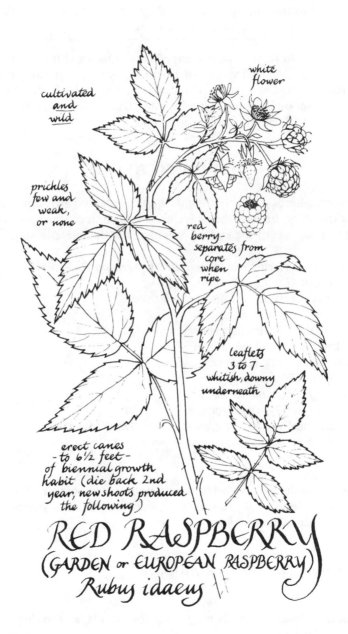

cultivated
and
wild

white
flower

prickles
few and
weak,
or none

red
berry-
separates from
core
when
ripe

leaflets
3 to 7 -
whitish, downy
underneath

erect canes
- to 6½ feet -
of biennial growth
habit (die back 2nd
year, new shoots produced
the following)

RED RASPBERRY
(GARDEN or EUROPEAN RASPBERRY)
Rubus idaeus

Late Pregnancy Tea. To make this tea, pour 1 cup boiling water over ½ teaspoon each of blue cohosh, squaw vine, raspberry leaf, and peppermint. The peppermint is used for energy, for flavor, and to prevent the nausea that sometimes occurs with blue cohosh. Cover and let steep for 15 minutes.

Drink one to three cups per day. While you are drinking this tea, you can discontinue your daily cups of raspberry leaf tea. If nausea occurs, or if you feel repulsed by this tea, eliminate the blue cohosh, and use an additional ½ teaspoon of squaw vine instead. During labor, drink up to three cups per day to facilitate contractions.

HERBS TO AVOID

The following herbs probably should *not* be used internally, especially during the first trimester, because they have been known to cause abortions (though some are used toward the end of pregnancy to facilitate labor).

Pennyroyal (*Hedeoma pulegiodes* or *Mentha Pulegium*)
Osha root (*Lilium filicinum*)
Blue cohosh (*Caulophyllum thalictroides*)
Black cohosh (*Cimicifuga racemosa*)
Squaw vine (*Mitchella repens*)
Spikenard (*Aralia racemosa*)
Cottonroot bark (*Gossypium hirsutum*)
Mistletoe (*Phoradendron serotinum*)
Tansy (*Tanacetum vulgare*)
Yarrow (*Achillea millefolium*)
Goldenseal (*Hydrastis Canadensis*) (Don't take more than ¼ teaspoon or one 00 capsule per day.)

The following laxative herbs should not be used because of their possible toxicity to the fetus, and because they can cause intestinal griping or spasms which can induce contractions.

Cascara sagrada (*Rhamnus purshianus*)
Buckthorn bark (*Rhamnus frangula*)

These herbs are generally too strong for infants, and so they may be too strong for the fetus.

Ephedra (There are various ephedra species. It is also known as desert tea, Mormon tea, or Ma Huang.) Ephedra speeds up the heart. Don't take more than ½ teaspoon of ephedra at a time, or more than ¼ teaspoon of the stronger Chinese ephedra, Ma Huang.

Echinacea (*Echinacea purpurea*). This herb can cause stomach upset in children. Don't take more than ½ teaspoon at at time.

Valerian (*Valeriana officinalis*). Valerian is a powerful sedative. Don't take more than ½ teaspoon at a time.

Mugwort (*Artemisia vulgaris*). All of the artemesias are cautioned against during pregnancy. Don't take more than ½ teaspoon at a time.

Cayenne (*Capsicum frutescens*). Many children are bothered by the extreme heat of cayenne. Don't take more than ⅛ teaspoon of powdered cayenne at a time.

Other herbs to avoid include the following:

Comfrey (*Symphytum officinale*). It would be prudent to avoid internal use of comfrey during pregnancy. Very small amounts of active cancer-causing compounds have been found by reliable sources. These compounds are found mostly in the roots, but some have been found in the leaves. External use is okay.

Coltsfoot (*Tussilago Farfara*). It would be prudent to avoid or minimize your use of this herb during pregnancy, since cancer-causing chemicals have been isolated from this plant. Rodents fed coltsfoot throughout their lifetime developed cancer.

Sage (*Salvia officinalis*) and desert sagebrush (*Artemisia tridentata*). Used to dry up the breast milk, they should be avoided, especially during the last trimester and while nursing. Desert sagebrush should be avoided throughout pregnancy.

Angelica (*Angelica Archangelica*). This herb is used to help expel the placenta by bringing on contractions.

Birthroot (*Trillium erectum*) (also called bethroot, or trillium). This herb is used to bring on labor.

Note: Several sources caution pregnant women against using slippery elm during pregnancy. This is unfortunate because it is an excellent remedy for gas and heartburn during pregnancy. It is one of the gentlest and mildest of herbs. The belief that slippery elm is an abortant dates back to when a midwife would insert a piece of slippery elm bark into the uterine os. It would work as a local irritant, which would then stimulate contractions, leading to an abortion.

FOOD AND DRUGS TO AVOID

Most pregnant women have a marvelous instinct about what they should eat. If you cultivate this intuition during pregnancy, you can carry it with you for the rest of your life. Pay attention to your body; indulge your cravings whenever possible — as long as the foods you crave are healthy.

Pregnant women shouldn't take anything that doesn't agreeably pass by their intuitive censors, the mouth and nose. If anything gives you a rush of nausea, try to avoid it. This includes herbs and other substances that are taken in 00 capsules, or as vaginal or rectal suppositories. The pregnant vagina absorbs much more easily than the nonpregnant vagina.

On the other hand, some substances may be rejected because their taste or smell is unfamiliar. Nutritional yeast is a good example. You may be repulsed by it at first, but after eating it a few times, you may develop a craving for it.

The fetus is forming its internal organs from the fifteenth day after conception (around the first missed period), until the end of the third month of pregnancy. During this time, be especially careful to avoid all drugs and toxic agents.

Even massage, including foot massage (reflexology), should not be too rough during pregnancy. Acupuncture should be done only by a master.

Try to avoid the following substances throughout pregnancy.

Caffeine

In 1980, the U.S. Food and Drug Administration advised pregnant women to avoid or minimize consumption of products containing caffeine. There appears to be an association between caffeine intake and birth defects. It may also be a cause of miscarriages, stillbirths, and low birth weight babies. Coffee is a diuretic; it makes you urinate more than usual so that vitamins B and C (the water-soluble vitamins) get washed out. These nutrients are particularly important during pregnancy. Coffee and other diuretics are harmful because they diminish the baby's blood supply.

Caffeine occurs naturally in coffee, black tea, and cocoa, and it is added to cola drinks. An average five-ounce cup of brewed drip-method coffee contains 115 mg. of caffeine. Percolated coffee contains about 80 mg., and instant coffee contains about 65 mg. An average cup of imported brewed black tea contains 60 mg. of caffeine, U.S. brands contain about 40 mg., and instant contains about 30 mg. One ounce of Baker's chocolate contains about 26 mg. of caffeine, semisweet dark chocolate contains 20 mg., milk chocolate contains 6 mg., and a cup of cocoa contains 5 mg. of caffeine.

Caffeine is also found in soft drinks. They contain anywhere between 58.8 mg. caffeine (in sugar-free Mr. Pibb) to 36 mg. (in Diet Pepsi).

Unfortunately, decaffeinated coffee may not be a good substitute. The usual high temperature roasting process for both caffeinated and decaffeinated coffee can create cancer-causing substances in the beans, and there are some indications that both regular and decaf coffee may contribute to bladder and pancreatic cancers. The main chemical solvent used in the decaffeination process is methylene chloride, a chlorinated hydrocarbon that has caused liver cancer in lab mice. It occurs in extremely low concentrations in decaf coffee. If you wish to avoid it, try Procter and Gamble's High Point coffee, which uses ethyl acetate — which occurs naturally in many foods, and is supposed to be safe. Nestle's Taster's Choice and Nescafe uses a "component occurring naturally in the coffee bean itself" but refuses to identify it. Specialty coffee stores carry other decaffeinated coffees prepared without methylene chloride.

Ultimately, the best solution may be to abandon coffee altogether. If you still crave the taste, try coffee substitutes, such as Inka, which is made from roasted rye, barley, chicory, and beet roots. It has a pleasant flavor reminiscent of coffee. These are available in most health food stores.

People crave coffee or soft drinks or chocolate because of the energy boost they get from the caffeine. A good habit to cultivate during pregnancy is drinking a Tigress Smoothie (see index) or having a Yogurt Delight (see index) when you want extra energy. The molasses and brewer's yeast will give you the energy you need, and plenty of nutrients as well.

Raw Meat
Eating raw meat is a possible source of toxoplasmosis (described later under "Kitty Litter").

MSG (Monosodium Glutamate) or Accent
This is used to give flavor to foods, especially in oriental cooking, and it is present in commercial soy sauce as a chemical additive. MSG was once added to many baby foods but was withdrawn when it appeared to cause brain damage in newborn babies of several animal species. The law requires it to appear on the labels of soups and canned goods, but not necessarily on the labels of salad dressings and mayonnaise.

Mineral Oil
Avoid products that contain mineral oil. Even external use is harmful, because this oil is absorbed through the skin, and then the fat-soluble vitamins (A, D, E, and K) dissolve in it and are carried out through the feces.

Massive Doses of Vitamin C
A reasonable amount of this vitamin is beneficial for pregnant women; but megadoses of 4,000 mg. per day during the first trimester can lead to abortion or possible birth defects. Also, taking massive amounts of vitamin C throughout pregnancy has been associated with creating a vitamin C dependency and even scurvy in newborns. I believe this can be explained by the fact

that taking high doses of vitamin C "teaches" the kidneys to excrete the vitamin at a high level. If the supplements are suddenly stopped, the kidneys will eliminate whatever natural vitamin C is being consumed, thus creating a deficiency. If you want to take megadoses of vitamin C during pregnancy, gradually decrease your vitamin C intake during the month preceding delivery, or give your newborn daily supplements of the vitamin.

Sodium Nitrate and Nitrite
These are common additives to luncheon meats and smoked meats and fish. Sodium nitrate can deform the fetus in pregnant women, and infants have died or been incapacitated from nitrite poisoning. Both substances are toxic at levels only moderately higher than the amounts used in food.

Aspirin (Acetylsalicylic Acid)
Try to avoid taking aspirin during pregnancy. It's particularly harmful during the last three months of pregnancy because it hinders absorption of vitamin K, which is necessary for proper blood coagulation. For this reason, it can result in blood coagulation complications in the newborn. It can also lengthen the duration of pregnancy and childbirth and can interfere with maternal blood clotting, making the possibility of hemorrhage greater.

If you must take aspirin, take one tablet of alfalfa with every tablet of aspirin, because alfalfa is high in vitamin K. While taking aspirin, be careful to avoid the simultaneous use of the following substances which can make aspirin even more harmful: benzoic acid (a common food preservative), alcohol (makes your stomach supersensitive to the irritating effects of aspirin, which can result in significant bleeding from the stomach wall), PABA (part of the B vitamin complex), and vitamin C (in sensitive individuals, it can intensify the effect of aspirin, resulting in side effects such as headaches and dizziness).

Aspirin is most commonly used for fever, pain, and inflammation. There are natural remedies for all of these conditions (see chapter 3). Tylenol (or any brand of acetamenophen) is just as effective as aspirin for fever and pain, yet it's virtually free of severe toxicity or side effects. However, it doesn't have the same anti-inflammatory action that aspirin has.

Antibiotics
Antibiotics tend to kill off the good flora in the body, along with the undesirable bacteria, and should be avoided whenever an effective substitute can be found. But there are times when it's better to take an antibiotic than suffer the consequences of a severe illness.

Some antibiotics affect the fetus more than others. For example, although penicillin does cross the placenta readily, it causes no apparent damage to the fetus. Tetracycline, however, is a specific antibiotic that should not be taken after the first four months of pregnancy because it can darken the baby's teeth and delay bone growth. Streptomycin has been known to cause deafness in the baby.

While taking any tetracycline antibiotic (including Tetracycline, Terramycin, Tetrex, Sumycin, Rondomycin, Robitet, Retet, Quidtet, Panmycin, Mysteclin-F, Declomycin, Cyclopar, Aureomycin, Achrostatin, and Achromycin), you should know that it will kill off good bacteria in your gut and will probably give you a stomachache. With this antibiotic, do not eat yogurt or other foods high in calcium within one hour before or two hours after taking tetracycline, because high calcium levels will drastically cut down on the effectiveness of this antibiotic. Wait until after you have finished taking the complete dose and then eat at least a couple tablespoons of yogurt three times a day or take an acidophilus tablet before meals, and eat foods high in calcium to help reestablish the beneficial bacteria. You can also insert a yogurt or acidophilus tablet in your vagina each night before going to bed. Continue this regimen for the same length of time that you took the tetracycline.

Avoid commercial bacon or luncheon meats cured with nitrites while taking Terramycin, because this combination has caused cancer in rats, and substances which cause cancer are believed to also cause mutations in developing babies.

Darvon (Propoxyphene)
Newborns can experience withdrawal symptoms if their mothers take this drug during pregnancy.

Valium (Diazepam)
This drug interferes with protein synthesis within the cells and prevents the normal growth of your baby's muscle cells.

Alcohol
The baby's blood alcohol level is equal to the mother's, but a baby has an immature liver and cannot handle nearly as much alcohol. If the mother consumes large amounts of alcohol, the baby may suffer from low birth weight, growth deficiency, poor sucking, cleft palate, irritability, hyperactivity, poor mental performance, convulsions, and withdrawal. It's possible that some of these abnormalities may be due to the poor nutrition of most alcoholics. Forty-four percent of the children of alcoholic mothers show some degree of mental retardation, and 32 percent have abnormalities of the head, face, limbs, and heart.

During the first days or weeks of pregnancy, the fetus is extremely sensitive to high concentrations of alcohol. Even just one evening of very heavy drinking during the early stage can result in abnormal babies. The use of alcohol during pregnancy has also been connected with spontaneous abortions and death of the baby shortly before or shortly after birth.

Marijuana

Comparisons of menstrual and hormonal functions of young women who use marijuana regularly show that 38 percent of the users suffered either from occasional cycles in which no egg was released or from shorter intervals of time between the end of ovulation and the expulsion of the endometrium – as compared to only 12 percent of non-users. And menstrual cycles of the users were an average of two days shorter than those of non-users.

Marijuana has caused cancer, mutations, and birth defects in the fetuses of lab animals. In experiments with rats who were given injected THC (the active property in marijuana) in doses roughly similar to what a human might consume, there were significantly more fetal deaths in the THC group than in the two control groups. Though the effect of injected THC is different than inhaling smoke, this study should make us cautious about the use of marijuana during pregnancy.

In the summary of the Fifth Annual Report to the U.S. Congress of the Health, Education and Welfare Department, 1975, the authors stated, "At this time, there is no conclusive evidence that the consumption of marijuana causes chromosome damage." Yet they expressed concern that there could be hormone-related adverse effects from the heavy use of marijuana during the first trimester of pregnancy. Since marijuana mimics estrogen, there could be abnormal sexual differentiation of the male fetus. Daily use of marijuana by the mother would give her an unusually high level of this female hormone. In fact, I do know of one woman who smoked marijuana daily throughout her pregnancy, and she gave birth to a boy with an abnormally tiny penis.

Unfortunately, there is little research being done on marijuana since there has been a decline in its use since 1979, but it is still by far the most widely used illicit drug. Long-term effects have not been verified. Yet it took a generation to establish the link between tobacco smoking and lung cancer. Another disturbing factor is that most previous and current studies are being done with marijuana that has a 2 percent THC content, while very potent marijuana is now being used which has a THC content as high as 14 percent.

LSD

The hallucinogenic drug LSD is an ergot derivative. Ergot is a fungus which occurs naturally in rye as small black particles. Ergot is removed from rye because it can bring on an abortion or premature labor by causing uterine contractions. I would suggest avoiding LSD while pregnant.

Cigarettes

Try to avoid cigarettes for as much as a year before conception. Women smokers have a 46 percent higher rate of infertility. They have a greater tendency to have irregular periods and abnormal vaginal discharge coupled with irregular vaginal bleeding. Studies have shown abnormally large areas of dead tissue on the placentas of women who currently or previously smoked.

A greater proportion of smoking mothers or former smokers have placenta previa—a condition in which the placenta is attached abnormally low in the womb, which can cause dangerous complications. There is also decreased sperm motility among men who smoke, so if you and your partner both smoke, you are likely to have trouble getting pregnant—especially if you are over thirty.

Every cigarette destroys about 25 mg. of vitamin C in your body and cuts down on your supply of oxygen. Vitamin C and oxygen are both vital nutrients for your unborn child. Babies born of cigarette-smoking mothers average six ounces lighter at birth. Low birth weight babies tend to be more fragile, and they may develop into youngsters who have a greater incidence of behavioral and learning problems.

Nicotine constricts the blood vessels, which limits the blood supply to the baby, which in turn diminishes the baby's supply of oxygen and nutrients such as iron, which are carried by the blood. The carbon monoxide from cigarettes crowds out the oxygen supply, so a woman who smokes two packs a day blocks up to 40 percent of her baby's oxygen. This may explain why miscarriages and spontaneous abortions are more common among women who smoke. Smoking over twenty cigarettes a day may stunt your baby's intelligence.

Your baby is twice as likely to be stillborn or to die soon after birth if you smoke cigarettes. And cigarette smoke also causes high blood pressure in newborns because of the poisonous cyanide.

Most pregnant women feel a natural repulsion to cigarettes. Listen to your body; this is a wonderful time to break a bad habit. However, if you absolutely must smoke, then please take the following vitamins for every five cigarettes you smoke (in addition to whatever amount you normally take): 25 mg. vitamin C, 20 I.U. vitamin E to increase your use of available oxygen, and vitamin K in the form of 1 alfalfa tablet to help prevent hemorrhaging during delivery and to protect against hemorrhagic disease in your newborn.

ENVIRONMENTAL HAZARDS TO AVOID

Kitty Litter Box

Cats are frequent carriers of the protozoa that causes toxoplasmosis. These organisms are constantly shed into the cat's feces where they become infectious to people after several days' incubation. Toxoplasmosis is characterized by the same symptoms as a common cold. Once a woman has toxoplasmosis, she is immune to it. But if a pregnant woman with no immunity is exposed to these organisms, the result may be infection of the fetus, causing extensive brain damage. Toxoplasmosis causes birth defects in one out of a thousand births.

Toxoplasmosis is more likely to occur when a woman who has never had a cat gets one when she is pregnant. A routine lab test, taken at the same time as the blood test for gonorrhea, will tell if you've had toxoplasmosis. If you haven't had it, you'd be wise to avoid getting a cat until after your baby is born.

Paint and Solvent Fumes
An old-fashioned method for inducing abortion was to have a woman paint a small enclosed room with oil-based paints.

Anesthetic Gases
A recent study revealed that almost 30 percent of the nurses working in operating rooms had miscarriages, in contrast to 9 percent of nurses working in other parts of the hospital. Gases used in hospital and dental anesthesia are a danger to pregnant women. The types of gases that have been implicated include nitrous oxides, halothane, and methoxyflurane.

Exposure to Pesticides
Miscarriages and deformities have been reported among women living in areas that have been sprayed with the herbicide 2,4,5-T or Silvex. In Vietnam 2,4,5-T was used in combination with 2,4-D and was known as "Agent Orange." Vietnam veterans who were exposed to these herbicides developed liver and kidney diseases as well as severe skin and nerve disorders. Some of their wives had miscarriages or gave birth to severely handicapped children.

Low doses of pesticides work more slowly and insidiously, but they are responsible for sterility, spontaneous abortion, birth defects, and mutations. In fact, low levels have the peculiar ability to escape the body's detoxification mechanisms, so that ultimately they can build up more toxic effects than massive doses. There is no level of dioxin that is free of toxic effects, and there is no antidote for it.

Radiation
Radiation sources include nuclear power plants, microwaves, x-rays, and video display terminals on computers.

Nuclear Power Plants. If the radioactive material from nuclear power plants leaks out — as it has already done in many locations — it gets into the water and the fish, into the grass and the vegetables, and it gets eaten by animals and people; then it gets into the meat and the milk, including human breast milk. If a baby drinks milk with radioactive iodine in it, or if a child eats fish or meat or vegetables contaminated with radioactive materials, these substances can get absorbed through the gut, and then go up to the thyroid gland in the neck where they will concentrate. They may irradiate just a few cells, and these cells may sit dormant for about fifteen years, and then suddenly go berserk and produce millions and billions of cells. The result is cancer.

Microwaves. Animal embryos subjected to microwave radiation show brain abnormalities and deformed spinal cords. Animals who graze under high-voltage power lines have stunted growth; animals and people living three hundred to five hundred feet away show changes in blood chemistry and electrocardiograms; at one thousand feet there are behavioral effects such as delayed reaction time.

Supposedly, there is no way to receive exposure from a microwave oven without bypassing several safety interlocks, and it is very easy to shield microwaves; a proper screen of thin metal foil is 100 percent effective in shielding all radiation. But, theoretically, if a microwave oven has a door leak, you could expose yourself by placing a part of your body in direct contact with the area. In this way, it is conceivable that after several hours you might receive a measurable exposure.

Developing embryos are vulnerable to the thermal effects of microwave radiation because they have little capacity to dissipate heat. However, I have found no research that indicates that microwave ovens have the capacity to produce mutations or malignancies.

But according to the late Dr. Hans Selye, the originator of the concept of stress, low levels of electromagnetic fields from sources such as microwave ovens and power lines can cause measurable biophysical stress responses in humans and animals.

X-Rays. Those who are most sensitive to the effects of radiation are fetuses, infants, and young children. Human beings get cancer more easily than any other animal on earth, and the youngest human beings are the most sensitive, since their cells are rapidly dividing and growing. Any radiation delivered to the trunk of either the mother or the father before conception can cause genetic damage, which may result in leukemia.

Infants exposed to x-rays in utero have a 40 percent increased risk of childhood leukemia, a 60 percent increased risk of cancer of the nervous system, and a 50 percent increased risk of all other cancers. If children of mothers who received x-rays while pregnant have not developed these diseases by the age of eight years old, their increased susceptibility levels out. Black children show no increased risk. The danger of x-rays in utero is particularly high for a fetus that is less than four months old.

People of child-bearing age should be careful to limit their exposure to radiation. If you must get x-rays while you are pregnant, or even if you suspect that you might be pregnant, insist on wearing a protective apron over your abdomen. Most technicians will be glad to cooperate. Any amount of radiation can be harmful, but dental x-rays and x-rays to the extremities are not known to cause any serious side effects.

Radiation is insidious because it can take fifteen or more years before its effects are seen, and by that time the cause has usually been forgotten.

If you are considering becoming pregnant (and are already trying to conceive) or are already pregnant, think it through very carefully before receiving any type of abdominal x-rays. X-rays taken for elective reasons should be delayed until after the pregnancy.

Computers. A video display terminal (VDT) is the part of the computer that looks like a television. In the process of creating an image on the screen the VDT emits various forms of radiation.

The media has reported at least eighteen documented clusters of adverse pregnancy outcomes among women who operate VDTs. In each of the reported clusters, a higher-than-normal rate of birth defects, spontaneous abortions, miscarriages, or stillbirths have occurred to clusters of women who operate VDTs in the same office. While the normal rate might vary from 14 to 20 percent of all pregnancies, in each of the eighteen reported clusters, the rate has ranged from 36 to 100 percent of the pregnancies in a single work location.

A women's group called 9 to 5 Working Women in Los Angeles set up a hotline to receive complaints about computer terminals. The group, which claims 12,000 members, said it had indications of fifteen new "clusters" of abnormal pregnancies in the United States.

A recent survey of 13,000 VDT workers done by the Japanese General Council of Trade Unions, discovered that about one-third of the 250 women who became pregnant or gave birth after working with VDTs had problems, including eight miscarriages, eight premature births, and five stillbirths. One might be tempted to dismiss this since there was no control group, and "problems" covers quite a broad territory. But the staggering fact was that the problems increased in relation to the time spent on VDTs. Two-thirds of those spending six or more hours per day on terminals had problems; 46 percent of those who spent three to four hours per day had problems; and 25 percent of those who spent less than an hour per day on VDTs had problems.

A Swedish study released in 1986 exposed pregnant mice to the kind of pulsed magnetic fields emitted by VDTs and found it caused severe defects in the fetuses. It showed that exposure of female mice during the first fourteen days of pregnancy to a pulsed magnetic field roughly comparable to a VDT produced an incidence of fetal malformations that was four to five times higher than the rate in the control group. Even more remarkable was the fact that three of the litters had two malformed fetuses, compared to nearly 900 recent controls in which this never occurred. They also found a greater incidence of birth defects, club foot, cleft palate, and eye and ear malformations.

One might ask why there is such a discrepancy between reports from the U.S. and reports from Japan and Sweden. In his excellent book, *Terminal Shock — The Health Hazards of Video Display Terminals*, Bob DeMatteo explains that attempts have been made in the U.S. and in Canada to introduce basic VDT health and safety regulations, but the computer industry has launched a multimillion-dollar campaign to defeat new legislation designed to protect VDT users. These groups formed a powerful lobby, the Coalition on Workplace Technology, which includes the American Newspaper Publishers Association and the American Bankers Association.

In 1984, newspaper offices used more than 50,000 VDTs. It is in their interest to keep the cost of VDTs to a minimum. The computer industry will sell more computers if the public is convinced that they are harmless, and if the price is kept low.

Meanwhile, when we have to consider the next generation, it is better to err on the side of being overcautious. Legislation is being introduced to enable VDT operators to change jobs while they are pregnant. In Canada, an Ontario labor arbitration board ruled that a VDT operator cannot be penalized for transferring to a non-VDT job during pregnancy. The board sensibly stated that people are entitled to be skeptical of scientists' conclusions, given the changing opinions about the safety of urea formaldehyde, DDT, 2,4-D, contraceptives, and other products.

If you are pregnant, or if you are trying to become pregnant, try to avoid using VDTs until after your baby is born.

If you must work, watch for side-effects. If you suffer from upset stomach, digestive problems, fatigue, sleeplessness, irritability, headaches, dizziness, ulcers, rapid heart beat, high blood pressure, or angina (chest pain), be sure to see your physician. However, these are not necessarily signs of exposure to radiation. They may simply be signs of stress due to the conditions under which you are working. Try to minimize the amount of time you spend on a VDT and observe the following guidelines, which will help to minimize your exposure to radiation and reduce the amount of physical stress.

1. Time Limit on VDT. Do not spend more than a maximum of four hours per day on the VDT. Every hour of work should be followed by a fifteen-minute rest period. During your break, move away from the VDT if it is still on. Walk around. Try to get some fresh air and sunshine. Get some exercise. Never work for more than one hour and forty-five minutes without a fifteen-minute break.

2. Lead Shielding. VDTs should have lead shielding to avoid radiation hazards. Terminals should be tested for radiation emissions.

3. Glare. Each VDT should be fitted with a nonglare screen, as well as a cover, hood, and brightness and contrast controls.

4. Location. If you are working in an office, and if the shielding is inadequate, you could be getting radiation just from being behind or alongside of someone else's VDT. Try to locate your work area at a distance from other computers.

5. Lighting. VDTs should be located away from windows. You should not be facing a window, nor should you have a window or bright light or even a white wall directly behind you. Windows should have blinds or drapes. Light sources should be adjustable.

6. Screen and Keyboard Position. The keyboard should be detachable and the angle should be adjustable. The screen should be eighteen to twenty inches away from your eyes.

7. Ventilation. You should have adequate ventilation in the room.

8. Chairs. The height of your chair should be adjustable, preferably while you are seated. The back of your chair should be adjustable and should provide support at the small of your back. Ideally, the back of your chair should be spring-loaded, so that it pushes gently against your back. If this is not available, try to obtain a chiropractic cushion which will support your back. Ask your local chiropractor about these. A foot rest is also a good idea.

9. Desks. Ideally, these should be adjustable for height of the keyboard, and wide enough to enable the monitor to be eighteen to twenty inches from your eyes.

10. Eye Exams. Have your eyes examined every year. If you wear glasses or contacts, consider getting special glasses or contacts to use while working at the distance required by the VDT.

11. Conductive Mesh Filters. These fit over computer screens and prevent the formation of an electromagnetic field, absorbing and safely draining radiation emitted through the screen. However, they do not screen out radiation that may be emitted from the rear, sides, bottom, or top of the VDT. These filters also reduce glare without reducing image resolution. Most people feel the difference in their eyes immediately. The filters are priced under $100.

SEXUALITY DURING PREGNANCY

Sexuality can be a sensitive area during pregnancy and while nursing. There is no medical reason why you should not be sexually active throughout pregnancy and lactation, except for the three-to-six-week-period directly after childbirth when the lochia (the bloody discharge) is still flowing.

Some women experience heightened sexual feelings during the middle months of pregnancy as the vaginal tissues become engorged and fetal pressure stimulates the genital organs. There's no reason why lovemaking should be harmful to either you or your child, provided that your partner is sensitive to what feels right to you. You should tell your partner what feels comfortable, and what doesn't. You may want to make love for shorter periods, or to lie on your side, or to be on top. Or you may not want to make love at all.

While you are pregnant and nursing your hormones may be so single-mindedly directed toward nourishing this new being that you may experience a loss of sexual desire. Many men experience a heightened need for loving during this time, when their mate seems to have the least amount of energy for them. This often results in them seeking other relationships.

During the last three months of pregnancy, if either you or your partner has a new sexual partner, it can endanger the baby, because of the possibility of contracting herpes, gonorrhea, a chlamydial infection, or AIDS. You could then pass this on to the infant, with serious or even fatal consequences.

THE FATHER'S ROLE IN PREGNANCY

When a couple is in love, they glow. When they decide to have a baby, they share the miracle of knowing that their love can create a whole new being. When their seeds join, the radiance rises and you may know that they are pregnant just by looking at their faces. I've known many men who have ripened along with their women, who shared their partner's agonies and joys, who gave massages and support all through the delivery, and who love and nurture their children just as tenderly as any mother.

A man who has a good relationship with his partner can give vitally needed emotional support. Dr. Monika Lukesch rates the quality of a woman's relationship to her spouse as the second most important factor in determining the physical and mental health of the child. (The first is how a woman feels about being a mother, and a man can have a strong influence on this, also.) Whether she feels happy and secure or ignored and threatened will have a decisive effect on her unborn child. On the basis of a study of over 1,300 children and their families, Dr. Lukesch estimates that a woman locked in a stormy marriage runs a 237 percent greater risk of bearing a psychologically or physically damaged child than a woman in a secure, nurturing relationship. She found that unhappy marriages produce children who are five times more fearful and jumpy than the offspring of happy relationships. At four or five years old, these children are undersized, timid, and inordinately dependent on their mothers.

If the mother of your developing baby is happy, then the chemistry of her body and the beating of her heart and the warm affection she feels toward you will penetrate and contribute to the sense of well-being that the baby experiences while inside her womb. For the majority of women, there is no other human being in the world who can make her feel as happy and good about herself as her mate can.

Stroking the Unborn

When your partner becomes pregnant, be sure to stroke her belly and speak to your baby. Studies have shown that the unborn child actually hears its father's voice in utero, and when a father has spoken soothingly to his baby before birth, the newborn is able to pick out his father's voice in a room. And if the baby is crying, the father's soothing voice can comfort the baby and help it to stop crying.

One midwife tells future daddies, "Play with your baby while he is still inside."

Your Health as a Father

Before conception, both the father and the mother should be in good health. Don't underestimate your role in the health of your child. The condition of your body at the time of conception will definitely affect the health of your baby. Any stockbreeder can tell you about the genetic importance of a strong, healthy bull or stallion.

Dr. Wilfred E. Shute showed in experiments with a group of fathers who had had babies with birth defects, that by giving the father vitamin E prior to conception of another child, there was only one abnormal baby—instead of the statistically expected seventeen.

Substances for Men to Avoid or Minimize

Babies are made from seeds. The seed comes from both the male and the female. Anyone who has a garden knows that healthy seeds tend to produce healthy plants. Your life-style—what you smoke, drink, and eat, and the environment in which you live—has a strong effect on your seed.

In the 1920s the average American male had a sperm count of 90 million sperm per milliliter of semen. By 1974, the average count had dropped to 65 million. A continuing downward trend has been shown by other studies in Japan and Europe. Semen is comprised of about 10 to 40 percent sperm cells. And yet several of the following substances, when used in extreme excess, have reduced the sperm count to zero!

Cigarettes. Some studies indicate that smoking has a direct effect on fertility by decreasing sperm motility; that is, the sperm can't swim hard enough and fast enough to reach their destination. Several studies have linked fathers who smoke with abnormal sperm, miscarriages, and birth defects. The frequency of birth deformities increased with the number of cigarettes smoked by the father, regardless of the mother's smoking habits, and the number of stillbirths was higher in families where the man smoked more than half a pack a day.

There are also indications of diminished production of the male hormone, testosterone, in heavy smokers. Some studies show that when the man smokes, it elevates the risk of having a lowbirth weight baby. These babies tend to be more fragile and have a greater incidence of behavioral and learning problems in later life.

Researchers found mutagens in the urine of smokers, but none in the control group of nonsmokers. Men who smoked more than thirty-one cigarettes a day ran a 100 percent higher chance of having mutations in their sperm than those who never smoked. These researchers concluded that smoking could have a serious impact on the gene pool of the entire human race.

Try to quit smoking at least one year before attempting to conceive. This will help to protect your child before and after birth, since children who live in the same home with a smoker are much more likely to get bronchitis, asthma, and other respiratory disorders.

Alcohol. Chronic use of alcohol reduces fertility in the male by causing an absence of sperm in the semen, as well as shrinkage of the testicles. There is also evidence that alcohol can inhibit the production of testosterone in the testicles. Continued intake of alcohol can result in permanent sterility.

Many men who consume large amounts of alcohol have powerful sexual desires, but cannot perform. More and more alcohol is needed to achieve an erection until ultimately a state of impotence persists even when the man is sober. Then irreparable damage has been done to the nervous system and there is little hope for recovery. When heavy drinkers notice the first signs of impotence, they should regard this as a warning sign and abstain from drinking altogether.

Your drinking can be psychologically damaging to your children, as evidenced by the growing number of Adult Children of Alcoholics. It is devastating for a child to grow up with a parent who drinks heavily. Children feel insecure and unloved even when their parents do love them, because their parent's behavior is always unpredictable. If you want to raise a family, give up or minimize your use of alcohol.

Marijuana. Daily smoking of marijuana for one month, or smoking a few times a week for several months, can reduce testosterone levels by one half, which puts it at a preadolescent level. When lab animals were given THC (the active ingredient in marijuana), they had difficulty conceiving. Daily smoking has been shown to cause reduced sperm counts. Marijuana causes the formation of abnormal sperm cells, which means that it could be a mutagen capable of causing deformities in offspring.

Aspirin. Among men who were hospitalized for analgesic abuse (taking very large amounts of aspirin, paracetamol, and phenacetin), few had become fathers while taking these drugs. Experiments with animals show that large doses of analgesics cause atrophy of the testicles and inhibition of the production of sperm.

X-Rays. If the father is exposed to radiation of the trunk before conception, this can increase the child's risk of getting leukemia (cancer of the white blood cells). This is because x-rays to the trunk can damage the cells that produce sperm.

Computers. Though there has been much publicity about clusters of adverse pregnancy outcomes among pregnant women using VDTs, not much mention has been made about men. And yet in one study, proportionately more birth defects were found among male VDT users' offspring. According to Dr. Arthur Frank, in a recent study sponsored by The Newspaper Guild, there may be an effect on male spermatogenesis. The male reproductive organs are far more sensitive to exposure because of their location outside of the body. Research by Ayme and Lippman-Hand in 1981 suggests that paternal exposure to low-dose radiation may elevate the risk of Down's syndrome and other adverse pregnancy outcomes.

Lead. This is a heavy metal that causes genetic changes in the male or female reproductive cells, with an increase in abnormally shaped sperm. The wives of men who are exposed to lead run a greater risk of miscarriage and the children of fathers exposed to lead run a greater risk of early infant mortality. Lead toxicity is associated with smaller family sizes. Lead exposure is common to workers in industries that produce batteries, ammunition, paint, and certain types of glass.

Anesthetic Gases. These are used in dentist's offices and hospital operating rooms. The wives of operating room technicians are almost twice as likely as wives of unexposed technicians to have spontaneous abortions and a higher incidence of birth defects. The gases that have been implicated include nitrous oxides, halothane, and methoxyflurane.

Birth Defects Related to Men

It was formerly believed that only the mother's age affected the occurrence of Down's syndrome, but it is now known that in one-third of the cases, the extra chromosome that causes this defect comes from the father. In a study done in 1984 in Scotland by Campbell and Ogston, the parents of 145 children with Down's syndrome were studied to find out what characteristics or habits of parents seemed to contribute to the likelihood of having a Down's child. The major factor that proved to be of importance was whether either parent had a significant number of illnesses before the conception of their

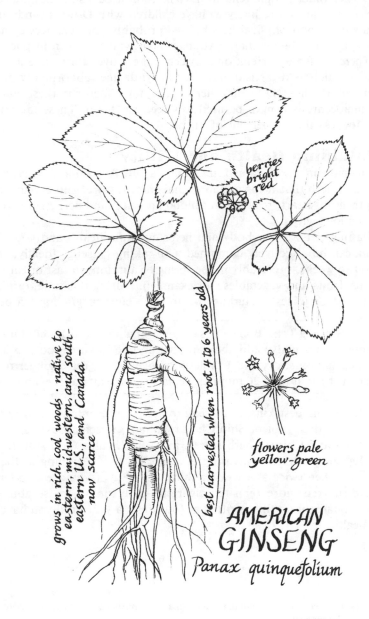

berries
bright
red

grows in rich, cool woods · native to
eastern, midwestern, and south-
eastern U.S. and Canada –
now scarce

best harvested when root 4 to 6 years old

flowers pale
yellow-green

AMERICAN
GINSENG
Panax quinquefolium

child. Since older people tend to have more illnesses, statistics indicate that older couples are more likely to have children with Down's syndrome. But if you are in good physical health, then probably your chances of having a healthy baby are better than a younger man who has been in poor health.

There is also a correlation between fathers over thirty-five and certain mutations such as dwarfism and Marfan syndrome (abnormality of height, vision, and the heart). The mother's age is not a factor in these conditions, and amniocentesis cannot be used to screen for them. These mutations account for less than 1 percent of births.

Maintaining Health and Virility

Ginseng has long been valued in China, Japan, Australia, Russia, and elsewhere as a herb that helps a man to maintain, restore, and enhance virility, strengthens his heart, regulates his blood pressure, and perpetuates youthfulness and longevity.

Fasting cleanses the body and helps maintain health and youthfulness. Fasting can be effectively combined with taking ginseng. Ideally, set aside one to two weeks, preferably in the spring or autumn, to fast or eat a simple diet (just fruits and vegetables, for example). During this time, drink plenty of teas and/or juices, including two to three cups of ginseng tea per day.

Ginseng Tea. Boil 6 cups of water in a pot. Add 1 medium-size root. You can also add about 1 tablespoon of licorice root, ½ inch of cinnamon stick, and 1 tablespoon of freshly grated ginger root. Simmer for at least 20 minutes, replacing the water as it evaporates.

Ideally, the best kind of ginseng to use for preventative and restorative purposes is Korea root or Shin Chu or Yi-Sun. Ginseng is available at most herb stores and Chinese herb stores, and some health food stores.

Men should follow this program once a year, beginning at the age of thirty, and then twice a year after thirty-five. But if you are in poor health or have smoked more than ten cigarettes daily or otherwise abused your health, you might do this as often as four times a year until you have rebuilt your health.

REFERENCES

Ernest L. Abel, Ph.D., "Smoking and Pregnancy," *Journal of Psychoactive Drugs*, 17, No. 4, (October-December) 1984.

Paavo Airola, N.D., *How to Get Well* (Health Plus Publishers, 1974).

"Amniocentesis Kills 1.5% of Fetuses in British Study," *Medical World News*, February 16, 1976.

Donna Day Baird, Ph.D., and Allen J. Wilcox, M.D., "Cigarette Smoking Associated With Delayed Conception," *Journal of the American Medical Association*, 253, No. 20, (May 24/31) 1985.

Steward Brand, "Human Harm to Human DNA," *CoEvolution Quarterly*, No. 21, (Spring) 1979.

Gail Sforza Brewer, *The Pregnancy-After-30 Workbook* (Rodale Press, 1978).

Irwin D. J. Bross et al, "Genetic Damage from Diagnostic Radiation," *Journal of the American Medical Association,* 237, No. 22, (May 30) 1977.

Helen Caldicott, M.D., "At the Crossroads," *New Age Magazine*, (December) 1977.

"Canadian VDT Ruling: No Loss of Pay for Alternative Work During Pregnancy," *Microwave News*, (March) 1982.

Center for Science in the Public Interest, *Chemical Cookery* (1977).

"Counseling the Pregnant Woman Exposed to Radiation and Estimating the Risks," *Current Problems in Pediatrics*, (September 14) 1984.

Paul Cressman, "Reproduction Under Siege," *Chimo*, (December) 1981.

Joan Davidson, "Singing the Low-Down Sugar Blues," *Chimo*, (December) 1981.

Adelle Davis, *Let's Get Well* (Harcourt, Brace and World, 1965).

Adelle Davis, *Let's Have Healthy Children* (Signet, 1972).

Bob DeMatteo, *Terminal Shock, The Health Hazards of Video Display Terminals* (New Canada Publications, 1985).

Do-It-Now Foundation, *Smoking, Drinking and Pregnancy*, DIN 108, (November) 1978.

Environmental Action Foundation, *Accidents Will Happen: The Case Against Nuclear Power* (Harper & Row, 1976).

"FDA Orders Propoxyphene Warning," *Health Newsletter*, (May) 1978.

"The Flap Over the Zap," *Newsweek*, July 17, 1978.

Arthur Frank, "Effects on Health Following Occupational Exposure to Video Display Terminals," a report from the Department of Preventive Medicine and Environmental Health, University of Kentucky (1983).

Tim Harper, "Marijuana: Pot Research Dwindling as the Drug Gets Stronger," *The Vancouver Sun*, May 17, 1986.

Carol J. R. Hogue, "The Effect of Common Exposures on Reproductive Outcomes," *Teratogenesis, Carcinogenesis, and Mutagenesis*, 4, No. 1, 1984.

John D. Kirschmann, *Nutrition Almanac* (McGraw-Hill, 1975).

W. R. Lee, "Working with Visual Display Units," *British Medical Journal*, (October) 1985.

"Librium and Other Common Drugs Tied to Cancer in Rats When Eaten With Nitrites," *Washington Post*, June 27, 1978.

Marijuana and Health, Fifth Annual Report to the U.S. Congress from the Secretary of Health, Education, and Welfare, 1975.

"Marijuana a Threat to Fetuses?" *Modern Medicine*, June 15-20, 1978.

Martindale, *The Extra Phramacopoeia*, 26th edition, edited by Normal W. Blacow (The Pharmaceutical Press, 1972).

John McDougall, M.D., and Mary McDougall, "The Latest Thinking on Protein," *Vegetarian Times*, August, 1984.

National Academy of Sciences, National Research Council. *The Effects on Populations of Exposure to Low Levels of Ionizing Radiation.* Report of the Advisory Committee on Biological Effects of Ionizing Radiations (BEIR Report), Washington, D.C., June 1976.

Pritchard & Macdonald, *Williams Obstetrics*, 15th edition (Appleton-Century Crafts, 1976).

Gerald N. Robenburg, *Compendium of Pharmaceuticals and Specialties*, 13th edition (Canadian Phramaceutical Association, 1978).

Laurel Robertson et al, *Laurel's Kitchen, A Handbook for Vegetarian Cookery and Nutrition* (Nilgiri Press, 1977).

"Roundtable: Genitourinary Infections," *The Female Patient*, 3, No. 2, (January) 1978.

Susan Stern, "A Guide to Worrying Intelligently About Having a Baby," *CoEvolution Quarterly,* 21, (Spring) 1979.

"Study Says Smoking Perils Baby Even If Halted Before Pregnancy," *The New York Times*, January 17, 1979.

"Unwanted Guests," *Processed World*, 14, 1985.

"Valium: A Danger During Pregnancy," *Health Newsletter*, May 1978.

"VDTs: Model Contract Provision," Service Employees International Union, AFL-CIO.

Thomas Verny, M.D., with John Kelly, *The Secret Life of the Unborn Child* (Collins Publishers, 1981).

"Video Display Terminals and Pregnancy," *FDA Drug Bulletin*, 14, No. 1, (April) 1984.

Janel P. Wallace, M.A., "Exercises in Pregnancy and Postpartum," *The Female Patient*, February, 1979.

Kay Weiss, "Marijuana as a Contraceptive," *CoEvolution Quarterly*, (Spring) 1977.

Phyllis S. Williams, R.N., *Nourishing Your Unborn Child* (Avon Books, 1982).

"Women's Group Says Birth Problems Linked to Use of Computer Terminals During Pregnancy," *Sacramento Bee*, February 17, 1984.

Chapter 3
Healing Yourself During Pregnancy

Most of the ailments discussed in this chapter are the common, ordinary problems of everyday life. A few are specific to pregnancy. During pregnancy you want to be particularly careful to avoid synthetically based, over-the-counter or prescribed drugs, unless they are absolutely necessary. Even aspirin is potentially harmful to the developing fetus.

This is the perfect time to discover natural remedies for whatever ails you. All of the following remedies have been used by many pregnant women, and are recommended by midwives and care givers. If you have ailments that are not covered in this section, please see my book, *Healing Yourself* (The Crossing Press), for natural remedies for common problems. Whenever you consider using a natural remedy that is not listed here, be sure to check the list of herbs to avoid in chapter 2.

ACHES AND PAINS

The following remedies are very helpful for tension, strains, back pain, and general soreness.

External Treatments
First, remember the good old reliables: the ice pack, hot water bottle, heating pad, whirlpool, and gentle massage. (Rough or deep massage and saunas should be avoided during pregnancy.)

We all need to be loved and pampered. When you are in pain, your body is crying out for attention. Don't be afraid to indulge yourself. One good remedy is a hot bath. The bathtub-in-every-home is a major contribution of modern civilization. Virtually every ache and pain will loosen its clutches while you are immersed in a hot bath. But for maximum effectiveness, there is an art to bathing.

Herbal Bath. A sweet-smelling herbal bath is a wonderful way to alleviate aches and pains, muscle cramps, tension, and even insomnia and headaches — it soothes away every tense spot in your body. But be careful: if you remain in the bath for more than twenty-five minutes, you might fall asleep in the tub.

> **Herbal Bath**. Cover ⅔ cup of linden flowers and ⅓ cup rosemary with 4 cups boiling water. Steep in a covered pot for 10 minutes. Strain and add to your bath water.

Hot and Cold Bath or Soak. This bath is more stimulating than the herbal bath, and it is a technique that can be used after the herbal bath if you would like to feel energized. Begin with a hot bath (with or without herbs), then allow one or two inches of water to escape and replace with cold water. Repeat this procedure until the bath water reaches a tolerably cool temperature. The cold water will increase your circulation and give you energy. Sit in the cool bath briefly and then emerge and rub your body briskly with a towel.

If the pain is in a small area, it can be soaked in a basin in tolerably hot water for about ten minutes, and then in cool water for three to five minutes. If you have the time, continue to alternate between hot and cool.

Tiger Balm, White Flower Oil, and Liniment. After the bath or soak, apply Tiger Balm, White Flower Oil, or liniment. These remedies are useful even if you don't have time for a bath or soak.

Tiger Balm is effective when there is intense pain in a small area. It can be rubbed into particular sore spots. It will relieve some headaches when rubbed into the temples. It can give relief to sinus pain when applied over the sinuses. It brings a sense of intense heat to the area within five to ten minutes after applying. It stimulates circulation and breaks up congestion.

Tiger Balm is a salve made from strong aromatic oils of camphor, menthol, peppermint, clove, and cajeput. (Cajeput is an oil from the East Indies; it contains methyl salicylate.) There are two kinds of Tiger Balm: red and white. The red is considerably hotter than the white, and works well on the back, chest, and extremities. The milder white is best for the face. Keep Tiger Balm out of reach of children, because camphor is poisonous when taken internally. Keep away from eyes and mucus membranes, because it causes a burning sensation. (To avoid accidentally rubbing my eyes with a finger that has been used to apply Tiger Balm, I use the fourth or fifth finger of my left hand.)

Tiger Balm is made in China and sold in many stores where Chinese items are found, as well as many herb and health food stores. It comes in small and large vials.

White Flower Oil is also from China and is similar to Tiger Balm, though it is even more penetrating. Since it is an oil rather than a salve, it can be easily used over a large area, though it works well in small areas. White Flower Oil is made from strong aromatic oils of menthol crystal, wintergreen, eucalyptus, camphor, and lavender.

Commercial liniments can be purchased at most drugstores and health food stores. Herbal liniments are made with alcohol and penetrating and warming herbs, which increase circulation to the area. Massage the sore area with liniment for five to fifteen minutes, up to four times a day, preferably after a hot soak or bath.

Liniment. If you'd like to make your own liniment, make it now, because it takes a week to make, and that's too long to wait when you're in pain.

Combine 4 tablespoons cayenne pepper, 3 tablespoons powdered myrrh, and 3 tablespoons goldenseal root powder. Cover with 2 cups vodka. Put a lid on the bottle, shake it well, and store it away from the sun. Shake the bottle once or twice a day for 7 to 14 days. On the last day, don't shake it; just pour out the liquid (not the sediment) into another bottle, and cork (or use a jar with a tight-fitting lid). Store away from the sun, preferably in a brown or green bottle. (Note: most herbalists begin their tinctures on or shortly after the new moon, and finish them before the full moon, because it is believed that the drawing power of the waxing moon helps to extract the active properties from the herbs.

Internal Treatments

Bach Rescue Remedy. I carry this remedy with me wherever I go; it's useful in any crisis, large or small. It's good for physical pain and for emotional trauma. This remedy enables people who are hurt to calm down and deal with their problems, both physically and emotionally. It's perfectly harmless and can be combined with any medications.

Place four drops directly under the tongue, or in ¼ cup of water or fruit juice. Repeat the dosage every ten to fifteen minutes as needed, and then gradually decrease the dosage. Often one dose is enough. If the person is unconscious, and if the remedy is in a base of alcohol (as it usually is), it can be put on the inside of the wrists, behind the earlobes, on the lips, or wherever the blood vessels are close to the surface, because the alcohol will be absorbed through the skin.

The Bach Rescue Remedy was formulated by Edward Bach, a British doctor who, at the turn of the century, became discouraged with trying to cure physical ailments without dealing with underlying emotional problems. Being something of a mystic, he gave up his successful practice in London and moved to the countryside where he began to induce in himself various states of emotional and physical illness. He then wandered over the hillsides, looking for a flower to bring his altered emotional state back into equilibrium. He found thirty-eight flowers, each for a different state of mind, and developed a method of preparing tinctures from these flowers. These tinctures may be used separately or in combination, according to the needs of the individual. The Bach Flower Remedies are not a substitute for therapy, or for working out real life problems; they simply bring a person into a more favorable state, from which they can better cope with their problems.

One particular combination of flower tinctures is called the Rescue Remedy, because it is ideally suited for emergency situations. The Rescue Remedy is made from the flowers of star of Bethlehem (for shock), rock rose (for terror and panic), impatiens (for mental stress and tension), cherry plum (for desperation), and clematis (for the far-away feeling that often precedes fainting and loss of consciousness).

Warning: *Do not attempt to make a tea from these flowers.* The Bach Flower Remedies are prepared by a special method which is described in *The Bach Flower Remedies* by Nora Weeks and Victor Bullen (C. W. Daniel Co. Ltd., Ashingdon, Rochford, Essex, England). These remedies are so dilute that they are harmless, whereas a tea made from these flowers could be toxic. All the remedies can be ordered from Ellon Bach, USA, Inc., PO Box 320, Woodmere, New York 11598. In Canada, order from Bach (Canada), Box 68, Station J, Toronto, Ontario M4J 4X8. You can order a one-ounce bottle of Rescue Remedy, or the full set of thirty-eight tinctures, which would enable you to make up your own combinations of remedies.

I know that the Bach Flower Remedies will seem strange to some people, and there will be skepticism about their effectiveness. Since experience is the best teacher, I urge you to try it yourself. I'd like to share one of my own experiences with you.

I knew a young woman who got pregnant unexpectedly, and decided to keep the baby. Two months later her husband was arrested on a serious drug charge and faced a long sentence because he had a previous record. He wanted to stay with his wife and child, so they went into hiding. After a while, they realized that it was unsafe for her to live with him, or to be with him when the child was born.

She was close friends with my neighbor, and so she gave birth at my neighbor's house, with a doctor who did home deliveries. The baby was born with so much gas that he could not nurse, and he cried constantly, and could not sleep. After two days, my neighbor came and asked me if there was anything I could do for the baby. At first I tried giving him slippery elm tea (which is good for gas) with an eyedropper. But he quickly spit it out. This made me think of the Rescue Remedy, which can be administered externally. It seemed appropriate to use this remedy since the emotional stress the baby's mother had been living under throughout her pregnancy might well be responsible for the physical discomfort her baby was now experiencing.

So I put a few drops of the remedy on his wrists, behind his ears, and on his lips. After about fifteen minutes, the child settled down, closed his eyes, and went to sleep. He slept for a couple of hours, and when he awoke his mother gave him another dose of the Rescue Remedy. After a short while, he was able to nurse. After that, he seemed to be quite normal and did not need any further doses.

Calcium. Calcium is an effective painkiller. When your blood calcium level goes down, your muscles tend to spasm. Calcium is a good remedy for muscle spasm, back pain, elbow pain, tendonitis, sprained shoulder, and leg cramps. It's also useful for the pains of childbirth and dental pain. Calcium is good for the nerves.

Doses range from 1,000 to 2,000 mg. of supplementary calcium per day. You can take one to two tablets of 250 mg. every two or three hours while the pain is intense. After the pain eases, one to three tablets per day is usually enough until the pain subsides. A soothing bedtime drink of warm milk with honey or molasses is rich in readily available calcium.

ANEMIA

Anemia is a deficiency in either the number of red blood cells or the amount of iron absorbed and carried by those cells. The hematocrit blood test is used to measure the number of red blood cells and the concentration of iron in those cells.

A low red blood cell count is usually an indication of anemia. The level normally falls during the early part of pregnancy, but it should never be allowed to drop too low. Women who experience very heavy menstrual flow before conception or bleeding during pregnancy are particularly susceptible to anemia. Anemia by itself is not dangerous, but it leaves the mother no reserves in case of excessive bleeding during childbirth. So a woman with a low red blood count may be advised against having a home birth.

If you're a vegetarian, your red blood cell count may be normally lower than a meat eater's, so a low count doesn't necessarily indicate that you're anemic. But be sure to tell your doctor that you're a vegetarian, and eat plenty of molasses and other iron-rich foods to build up your reserves.

When the hematocrit is low, iron salts are usually prescribed, but iron salts interfere with the absorption of vitamin E in your intestines. Since vitamin E is important for the optimal use of oxygen, the iron salts indirectly diminish the baby's oxygen supply, which can result in miscarriage or premature or delayed birth, or other damage to your baby. Iron salts and vitamin E should not be taken at the same time. If iron salts must be taken, it's advisable to supplement the diet with at least 100 I.U. of vitamin E. The vitamin E can be taken in the morning, with breakfast or some form of fat, and the iron salts can be taken twelve hours later, after the vitamin E has been absorbed. Ferrous fumarate or gluconate are preferable to ferrous sulfate or chloride, which are very harsh on your body.

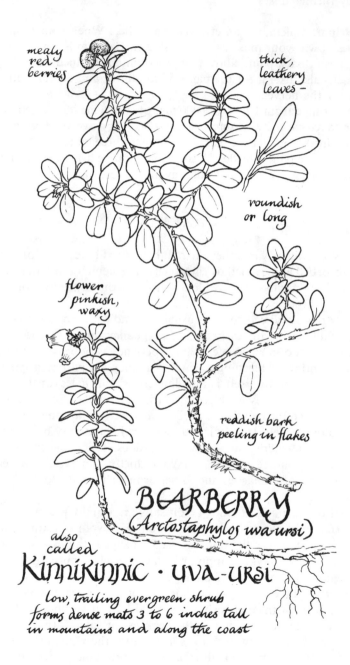

mealy red berries

thick, leathery leaves –

roundish or long

flower pinkish, waxy

reddish bark peeling in flakes

BEARBERRY
(Arctostaphylos uva-ursi)

also called
Kinnikinnic · uva-ursi

low, trailing evergreen shrub
forms dense mats 3 to 6 inches tall
in mountains and along the coast

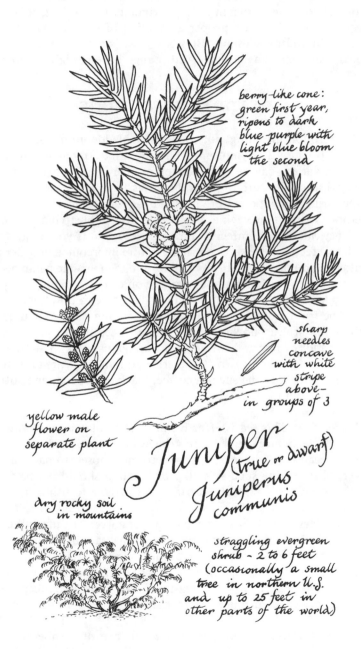

berry-like cone:
green first year,
ripens to dark
blue-purple with
light blue bloom
the second

sharp
needles
concave
with white
stripe
above—
in groups of 3

yellow male
flower on
separate plant

Juniper
(true or dwarf)
Juniperus
communis

dry rocky soil
in mountains

straggling evergreen
shrub - 2 to 6 feet
(occasionally a small
tree in northern U.S.
and up to 25 feet in
other parts of the world)

There are natural ways to build up your body's supply of iron, but it's not enough just to eat foods that are high in iron, because iron is difficult to absorb. If your diet is rich in iron and vitamins C, B6, B12, folic acid, and magnesium, this will insure proper absorption of iron. Molasses is a good source of iron and magnesium. Brewer's yeast is a fine source of B6, B12, folic acid, iron, and magnesium. And orange juice is high in vitamin C.

BLADDER INFECTIONS

If you have trouble urinating, you may have a bladder infection, but it's hard to diagnose because the symptoms – burning urine, frequent urination, and pain in the bladder – can be an indication of many things, including venereal or kidney disease. Be sure to get a diagnosis from a doctor.

Since urine is a good culture medium for bacteria to grow in, and since the urethra is close to the vagina, women are susceptible to bladder infections because they can become infected during intercourse. If you're prone to having bladder infections, be sure to urinate before intercourse in order to make that culture medium less readily available, and then urinate again after intercourse in order to wash out the bacteria. You can also dilute your urine by drinking at least eight glasses of liquid per day. After a bowel movement, be sure to wipe from front to back to avoid contaminating your urethra.

When you are run down, you are more susceptible to getting an infection, so get a lot of rest and cut down on strenuous work. You might try an alkaline diet for a week or two, as described on under "Vaginal Infections." Avoid drinks with caffeine such as coffee, black tea, cocoa, and soft drinks. Also avoid alcohol.

Bladder Tea. This tea is effective in treating bladder infections. Note, however, that echinacea and yarrow have been cautioned against during pregnancy because they have been known to cause upset stomach in children. However, when used in such a small proportion, it should not be distressing to your growing baby – and it is certainly preferable to using strong drugs.

Bladder Tea. Drink 1 cup per day for a week. To make the tea, bring 3½ cups water to a boil and add echinacea root. Simmer, covered, for 20 minutes, then remove from the heat and add 1 teaspoon yarrow flowers, 1 tablespoon bearberry (uva-ursi), 1 tablespoon corn silk (from Indian corn), and 1 teaspoon juniper berries. Steep for 15 minutes in a covered container, then strain. Store in the refrigerator.

Cranberry Juice. Drink at least one half cup of cranberry juice four times a day. Cranberry juice is especially good for cleaning out the kidneys and bladder. If you don't like cranberry, try cranapple juice.

Vitamin C. Take 1,000 to 3,000 mg. of vitamin C per day to make your urine acidic so that bacteria will not grow in it.

BURNS AND SUNBURNS

Always begin by cooling the burn with cold water or ice water until the burning sensation stops.

For a more serious burn, cool it and then take a piece of gauze and spread aloe vera, honey, vitamin E, or calendula cerate on the gauze and apply it to the burn. Secure the gauze with adhesive tape. Do not try to apply directly to the burn because that is much more painful to the fragile tissue.

If the burn is severe, consult a first aid manual and/or a doctor. Consider treating for shock (elevate legs, maintain body temperature with blankets) and give fluids if the person is conscious.

Sunburns are minor burns that can be prevented by limiting your early exposure to the sun to periods of ten or fifteen minutes, extending them gradually until you have a good tan. Use suntan lotion with a sun block.

Aloe Vera. This succulent plant yields an excellent ointment for all kinds of burns. Cut off a piece of the lower leaf (so that it will continue to put out new upper leaves), peel back the outer layer, and apply the thick jelly directly to the burn. In most cases, the effect is immediate: the redness can literally be seen going away and the pain eases at once. It can be used effectively for ordinary burns, and even for chemical burns and for radiation burns. The gel is bottled and sold, but it's best when taken directly from the plant. Aloe grows in indirect sunlight and needs watering only every seven to ten days.

Raw Honey. Raw honey is an excellent pain reliever. The skin absorbs the honey quickly, and the stickiness does not remain.

Vitamin E. Vitamin E is available in salves and ointments. Probably the most potent form, and the form which is most effective for burns, is the vitamin E oil that comes in capsules. The capsule can be pierced by putting a pin through both ends, and then the oil can be squeezed onto the burn. Be sure to wait until the burn has cooled, because if the oil is applied while the burn is still hot, the oil cooks on the skin, making it even more painful. Vitamin E is well known for its ability to prevent or eliminate scarring. When a deep burn occurs, the tiny blood capillaries are injured, and oxygen can't get to the cells. Scar tissue forms in the absence of sufficient oxygen. Vitamin E is a biological antioxidant, which means that it slows down the oxidation of fats in your blood and thereby maximizes your body's use of oxygen, which helps to prevent the formation of scar tissue.

Calendula Cerate or Salve. Although this remedy is not always readily available, it is my favorite for burns because it takes away the pain immediately, and you can easily carry it with you. Calendula cerate is a salve made of pot marigold flowers in a bland base. It's excellent for burns, sunburns, chapping, dryness, and diaper rash. A one-ounce tube lasts a long time and can be ordered at a reasonable price from Standard Homeopathic Company, PO Box 61067, Los Angeles, California. Or you can make your own salve.

Calendula Cerate. Heat 1 cup of vegetable oil (olive oil is a good base) until the first bubbles form, then add ¼ cup of dried or ½ cup of fresh pot marigold petals. Cover and keep the heat very low for 30 minutes. Then strain out the petals and slowly melt in ¼ cup of beeswax, cut into small pieces. When the wax is melted, remove from heat and add the oil of one capsule of vitamin E and ¼ teaspoon tincture of benzoin (available from drugstores) as a preservative. Pour into suitable containers; it will harden as it cools.

COLDS

A cold is not altogether a bad thing. I've learned to see it as a friend who comes to warn me that I've been working too hard and neglecting my body. It puts me to bed where I can drink nourishing teas and juices and allow my subconscious dream-mind to take over for a while so that my rational mind can rest.

I used to think I was clever: A cold would come and I would drink my teas and take my vitamins and continue working. I never got sick enough to go to bed, but the cold would hang on for weeks.

Now I can feel when I'm starting to get overworked; I can predict when the symptoms will start to set in. It may be a slight sore throat or sniffles or just a feeling of exhaustion. If I listen to the signals, I'll go directly to bed. I might just sleep in for a morning, or I might take the whole day off and set myself free from the workaholic bandwagon. If I do this, I don't get sick.

Some people just can't give themselves permission to have a good cry— so they'll have a head cold instead.

If your body is starting to send you signals, and you can't relax and have yourself a good cold, you may be able to meet your body halfway. By using any of the following procedures, together with getting more rest, a good diet, and enough exercise, you can usually strengthen your body's self-defense system and prevent a full-blown cold.

Cold Prevention

These are the most popular natural methods for preventing a cold, but they must be taken at the very first signs: a little mucus, a slightly sore throat, a cough, or a sneeze. If you wait a day or two, "just to make sure it's really a cold," it will be too late.

Vitamin C. At the first symptoms of a cold, begin taking 250 mg. of vitamin C every hour for up to twelve hours per day. If you get a cold at all, it will probably be very mild and won't last more than one or two days. Continue taking the same dosage of vitamin C until the symptoms subside, and then reduce the dosage gradually (for example, if you were taking 250 mg. six times per day, take it four times a day, and then twice a day).

Garlic. When the symptoms of a cold appear, eat one to two cloves of raw garlic, two or three times a day until the symptoms are gone—and then for two or three more days. Some people chop it up and add it to an oil and vinegar salad dressing; some crush it and add it to the butter on their toast. It's good mixed with yogurt and grated cucumber, or added to cooked chicken soup. Chew it raw, chop it up and swallow it down with water or tea.

To avoid the garlic smell, try kyolic garlic. It's more expensive, but it's available in capsules, and it's odorless.

About one in twenty people seem to be allergic to garlic. These people usually develop a stomachache or gas whenever they eat it. Eating yogurt or acidophilus will give relief, but use another remedy if garlic affects you this way.

Garlic and Lemon Tea. This tea tastes good, even to small children and to people who don't savor the taste of garlic.

Cut one clove of garlic into tiny pieces and put it in the bottom of a cup and squish with a spoon. Add the juice of ¼ small lemon. Put 1 teaspoon of mint or peppermint in the cup and pour in the boiling water. Cover and let brew for 3 to 5 minutes. Use honey as desired.

Hot Cider Vinegar and Honey Tea. This is a very convenient remedy when you're traveling because the ingredients can be found in almost every home and many restaurants. It tastes a bit like hot lemonade. Drink one to two cups per day.

Hot Cider Vinegar and Honey Tea. Put 2 tablespoons each of apple cider vinegar and raw honey in a cup and cover with boiling water. Stir and drink.

Cold Treatments

If your body does catch that cold—or if you decide that the time is right to go ahead and have it—follow these basic guidelines:

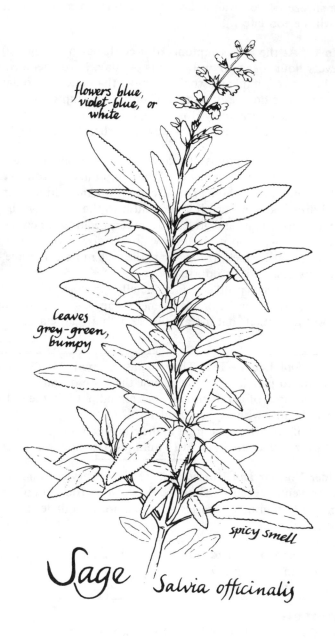

flowers blue,
violet-blue, or
white

leaves
grey-green,
bumpy

spicy smell

Sage Salvia officinalis

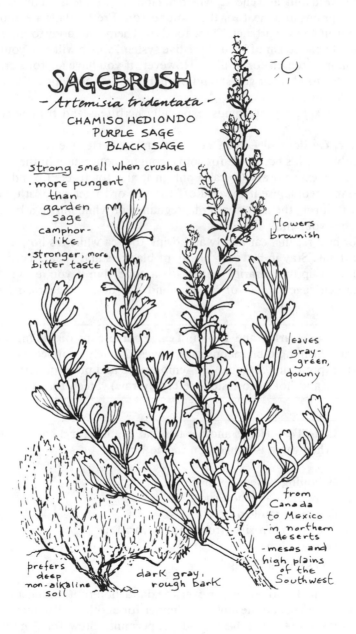

SAGEBRUSH
- Artemisia tridentata -

CHAMISO HEDIONDO
PURPLE SAGE
BLACK SAGE

strong smell when crushed
• more pungent
   than
   garden
   sage
camphor-
   like
• stronger, more
bitter taste

flowers
brownish

leaves
gray-
green,
downy

from
Canada
to Mexico
- in northern
   deserts
- mesas and
high plains
   of the
Southwest

prefers
deep
non-alkaline
soil

dark gray,
rough bark

1) Go to bed and get as much rest as possible. If you've been overworking, stop working entirely for at least a day, or until your body feels renewed.

2) Avoid milk and cheese, which are mucus-producing. You may want to eliminate grains and meat for the same reason. Fresh salads are good to eat. Or try a fruit and yogurt diet. These foods will help your body to eliminate toxins and take the strain off your digestive system, which will give your internal organs more strength for healing. However, if you have a strong craving for a particular food, then you should probably eat it—provided it's nutritious.

3) Avoid taking aspirin.

4) Drink plenty of liquids, especially herb teas and fruit juices.

Sage, Garlic, and Lemon Tea. This is very effective for upper respiratory problems. It's been used for colds, coughs, congestion of the sinuses and lungs, as an expectorant (to raise phlegm), and for fevers (to induce sweating). Many people use it to ward off the flu, or to get rid of it quickly. Do not use it during the last month of pregnancy or while nursing, because sage diminishes your milk supply.

For best results, eat lightly and drink the tea while it's hot, at least one cup per hour. Stay in bed with plenty of blankets and sweat. Your temperature may go up temporarily, but this is a good sign if you're sweating. Use only garden sage (*Salvia officinalis*) and not desert sagebrush (*Artemisia tridentata*).

Sage, Garlic, and Lemon Tea. Pour 6 cups of boiling water over 2 heaping tablespoons sage leaves, 2 finely chopped cloves of garlic (preferably organic), ½ lemon juice and pulp (preferably organic), and honey to taste (preferably raw). Steep for 5 minutes.

Lung Tea. Here's another tea that is good for a cold, particularly when there is congestion in the lungs.

6 cups boiling water
2 tablespoons dandelion root
2 tablespoons mullein
1 tablespoon corn silk (from Indian corn)
1 tablespoon lobelia
1 tablespoon peppermint

Pour the boiling water over the dandelion root. Simmer for 10 minutes, then add the mullein. Simmer for another 10 minutes, then add the corn silk, lobelia, and peppermint. Brew for 5 minutes. Strain.

Chicken Soup. Since time immemorial, mothers have given this soup to their sick children. People used to think it was just an easily digested food. But now chicken soup has been raised to its proper status as a true remedy for colds by a study at the Mt. Sinai Hospital in Miami, Florida, which showed that chicken soup speeds the expulsion of germ-laden mucus from the nasal passages.

Chicken Soup. Here's my mother's recipe (and it's a good one, whether you're sick or not).

1 whole chicken
3 potatoes
3 large carrots
2 onions
3 celery stalks with leaves
3 garlic cloves
1 tablespoon salt
2 teaspoons onion salt
2 teaspoons garlic salt
1 teaspoon poultry seasoning
1 teaspoon sage powder
1 teaspoon celery salt
⅓ cup barley

Wash the chicken in cold water. Place it in a pot and cover with water, then boil for 3 minutes, until the liquid becomes foamy. Skim off the foam. Chop the vegetables and add to the soup along with the seasonings and barley. Simmer for 2 to 3 hours, until the chicken falls off the bones. Remove the bones. Eat as much as you like.

Chest Congestion

Dry air (lack of humidity) is a prime offender in aggravating this condition. Wood or gas stoves and radiators should have a pot of water on them to keep the air from drying out. If you suffer from frequent congestion, a cold mist humidifier is a good investment. Vaporizers can be used as well, but they give off hot moist steam, whereas cold mist humidifiers give off a more effective cool mist.

Eucalyptus Steam. This is a popular, old-fashioned, and effective remedy. Add one teaspoon of eucalyptus oil (which can be purchased in any drugstore) to the water in a cold humidifier or vaporizer (the manufacturer's instructions may say not to add anything to the humidifier, but I have been doing this for years and have had no problems—just wash the humidifier after each use). Leave it on all night in a closed room. If you don't have a hu-

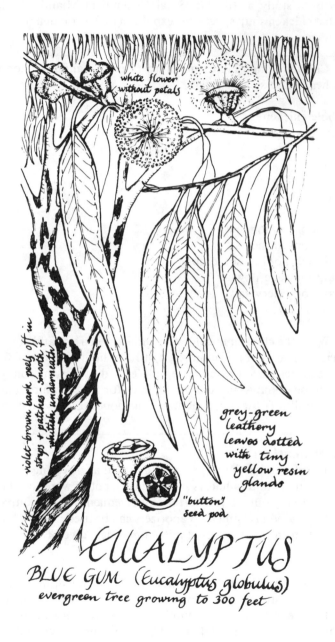

white flower without petals

violet-brown bark peel off in strips + patches - smooth + whitish underneath

grey-green leathery leaves dotted with tiny yellow resin glands

"button" seed pod

EUCALYPTUS

BLUE GUM (Eucalyptus globulus)

evergreen tree growing to 300 feet

midifier or vaporizer, you can just add the eucalyptus to a pot with one or two cups of boiling water. Remove the pot from the fire, put your head over the pot, cover your head with a towel, and inhale the fumes. (You'll have to come up for air a few times.) Even just opening up the bottle of eucalyptus oil and inhaling the fumes from the bottle can be helpful.

If you have access to a eucalyptus tree, you can use about six eucalyptus leaves and six seed pods in two or three cups of water. Simmer for ten minutes, then inhale as above. This water can be saved and used again several times until it loses its strength.

Tiger Balm. This ointment is good to rub on your chest and the upper back when you have chest congestion. See under "Aches and Pains" for more information on Tiger Balm.

Ginger. You can chew on a small piece of raw ginger or make a tea. It tastes hot and very soothing and also helps relieve head colds and sore throats.

> **Ginger Tea**. Grate 1 tablespoon whole fresh ginger. Boil 1½ cups of water, add the grated ginger, and simmer for 10 minutes. Strain and add honey if desired.

Coughs
Coughs respond well to the herbal remedies described below. Use as needed.

Honey and Lemon Juice. This is the most popular remedy for coughs. Honey soothes the mucus membranes by coating the throat and air passages. It's also high in potassium. Lemon juice is astringent; it causes the tissues to contract, reducing inflammation and swelling. It also cuts mucus and is high in vitamin C. Mix one tablespoon raw honey with the juice of half a lemon. Sip a teaspoon every hour and after a coughing spell.

Sage, Garlic, and Honey Tea. Sage will bring up mucus, relax the nerves, and stop coughing. It's also good for fever and other cold symptoms. (Look for the recipe under "Cold Treatments." Do not take during the last month of pregnancy or while nursing because sage diminishes breast milk.

Fever
There is a fever if the temperature (which should not be taken immediately after extreme physical activity) is 100 degrees F. (38 degrees C.) or more by mouth. During a fever, drink more than normal amounts of fluids, since the fever is literally burning up your body's moisture.

Avoid aspirin. Although health care givers do prescribe acetaminophen, there are natural methods for treating fevers which are very effective.

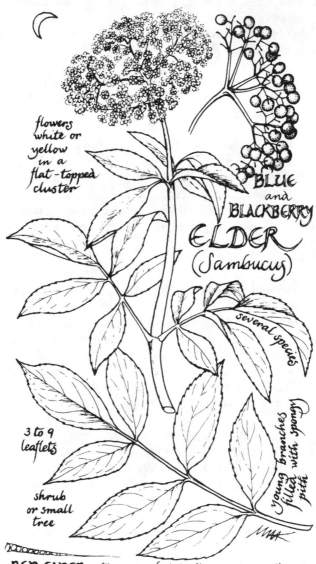

flowers
white or
yellow
in a
flat-topped
cluster

BLUE
and
BLACKBERRY
ELDER
(Sambucus)

several species

young branches filled with spongy pith

3 to 9
leaflets

shrub
or small
tree

RED ELDER - stronger, can be toxic; flowers not generally used

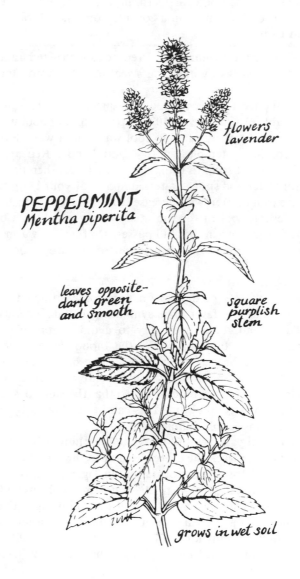

flowers
lavender

PEPPERMINT
Mentha piperita

leaves opposite-
dark green
and smooth

square
purplish
stem

grows in wet soil

Peppermint and Elder Flower Tea. This is a time-honored herbal treatment for fever which rarely fails. It usually takes effect within a couple hours or overnight.

> **Peppermint and Elder Flower Tea**. Boil 2 cups of water and pour over 2 tablespoons peppermint and 2 tablespoons elder flowers. Steep for 15 minutes in a covered container. Strain. Drink hot and go to bed.

Sage, Garlic, and Lemon Tea. Prepare as instructed under "Cold Treatments." This tea works by inducing sweating. Drink hot and go to bed.

Cooling the Heat. This method is frequently used in hospitals. If a fever is uncomfortable or if it exceeds 102 degrees, tepid or cool water can be used to bring it down. Start by running cool water on a washcloth and applying it to your forehead, temples, wrists, and hands. Repeat this every five minutes. If it doesn't seem to bring down the fever, then lie in a shallow tub of lukewarm water and sponge alternate parts of your body and extremities. The moisture evaporation will increase heat loss from your body. When you become chilled, get out of the tub, and wrap yourself in a blanket, but do not rub. Begin again when the chill passes. Do this in a warm (not hot) room with no drafts. Discontinue if your temperature drops too quickly.

Nasal Congestion

The mucus membranes of the nose may become inflamed due to a cold or an allergy, such as hay fever. The symptoms include a runny or stuffed-up nose, sneezing, and runny eyes. Try to avoid commercial nose drops or sprays which relieve by constricting the blood vessels and shrinking the swollen mucus membranes. After about three days, the blood vessels lose their ability to constrict and the symptoms are worse than ever.

It's helpful to keep the mucus thin so that the sinus passages and the eustachian tubes don't get plugged. This can be facilitated by drinking lots of fluids and by using a cold humidifier.

To open nasal passages and facilitate breathing, it's good to apply Tiger Balm to the area between the eyebrows and to the temples and earlobes (see "Aches and Pains" for more information on Tiger Balm). It also helps to add one teaspoon of eucalyptus oil to the water in a cold humidifier.

For dry nasal passages, apply one of the following with a cotton swab: vitamin E oil (just open a capsule of vitamin E with a pin and squeeze out the oil), vegetable oil (any kind will do, as long as the smell is agreeable), or calendula cerate (described under "Burns and Sunburns").

Sore Throat (Viral)

Sore throats caused by viruses often accompany a common cold, and the easiest way to cure them is by following the vitamin C or garlic therapy described under "Cold Prevention." The vinegar and honey tea described under "Cold Prevention" can be used as a gargle. Viral sore throats, like colds, go away on their own. About 90 percent of sore throats are viral. But viral infections cause the white blood cell count to drop, which makes you more vulnerable to other infections since white blood cells are the major combatants in fighting off disease. Home remedies will help relieve the symptoms and speed recovery.

If your sore throat lasts more than three days, or if — by looking at the throat with a flashlight — it's *very* red, particularly if there are white spots, or if there's a fever of 103 degrees or more, you may have strep throat. The test for strep is a simple throat swab, taken with a long Q-tip. It only takes a minute, and if your doctor or local clinic is cooperative, you should be able to come in just for a throat culture. These cultures are then sent to a laboratory, and it takes about twenty-four to forty-eight hours to get the results, so don't wait until you're dying before you go in for a culture.

Warm Salt Water Gargles. Add ¼ teaspoon salt to ¼ cup water. Gargle three to ten times every two to three hours. Most doctors suggest doing this. Salt shrinks inflamed tissue, and it helps to prevent a viral sore throat from turning into a bacterial strep infection. The salt solution causes the rigid cell walls of any invading strep bacteria to break down by osmosis and dehydration.

Vitamin C as a Throat Lozenge. Place a 250 mg. pill of rose hips or a 100 mg. pill of ascorbic acid in the back of your throat keep it there until it dissolves. Repeat every hour as needed.

CONSTIPATION

During pregnancy, the body produces high levels of progesterone which cause relaxation of the smooth muscles. This affects your intestines by reducing their motility. As the fetus in your belly grows larger, your stomach and intestines are displaced and compressed. Peristalsis (intestinal contractions which aid digestion) is slowed down and food remains in your stomach longer. Your stomach secretes less hydrochloric acid and pepsin, which are important in the breakdown of proteins. All of these factors combine to slow down digestion, contributing to constipation, which is a common complaint during pregnancy.

Only the gentlest natural laxatives are safe to use when you're pregnant. *Never use more than one remedy per day*, especially during your last trimester, because they can cause griping and cramping, which can then set off contractions, resulting in premature labor. If your due date is approaching and you have been constipated, you may want to change your diet and take a mild laxative to get your bowels moving before you go into labor. Otherwise you will probably need to use an enema while you are in labor.

The following remedies have a gentle laxative effect.

Dietary Remedies

Bran. This is by far the most popular remedy for constipation. Many long-standing, chronic cases have responded to it beautifully. It's a food, and so it works gently, without irritating the colon. Bran has a remarkable capacity to absorb moisture; when it's taken with plenty of liquid, it swells up and forms a soft mass that passes easily through the intestines. Raw or crude bran can be purchased in health food stores. It's preferable to packaged commercial bran cereals which contain less than one-third the fiber content and none of the moisture-absorbing properties of raw bran. Remember to drink plenty of liquid (one to two cups) at the same time.

People report taking anywhere from two tablespoons to one cup of bran per day. Many like to mix it with orange juice, or cereal, or bake it in muffins or pancakes.

Bran Muffins. These muffins make a delicious snack or a small meal, and they're high in nutrients that are essential during pregnancy.

2 cups whole wheat flour
1½ cups bran
2 tablespoons brown sugar (optional)
¼ teaspoon salt
¼ teaspoon baking powder (without aluminum)
1¼ teaspoons baking soda
2 cups buttermilk
1 beaten egg
⅓ cup molasses
¼ cup vegetable oil
1 cup raisins.

Preheat the oven to 375 degrees F. Combine and mix in one bowl the flour, bran, sugar, salt, baking powder, and baking soda. In another bowl, combine the buttermilk, egg, molasses and oil. Combine the contents of both bowls and mix with a few strokes, then add the raisins. Mix just until all the dry ingredients are wet. To prevent the muffins from sticking to the tin, combine 1 tablespoon vegetable oil and few drops of liquid lecithin and brush this onto the muffin tins (a pastry brush can be used). Pour the batter into the prepared tins and bake for 25 minutes.

Water. Constipation is often caused by insufficient fluid, so the stools get hard and dry. Coffee and beer do not count as fluids, because they're diuretic and cause you to lose fluid. Juices and herb teas are good, but water is best. Try to drink eight or more cups (two quarts) per day.

Raw Greens. This is an important part of the diet; greens contain lots of roughage. Try to eat one or two salads per day.

Prunes or Prune Juice. This traditional remedy for constipation is easily obtained and often works well. Use as needed. Start with one cup of juice, or a half cup of prunes per day, and increase until you get the desired result. Stewed prunes are quite tasty. Barely cover with water and add a touch of lemon juice and stew for about twenty minutes. Add other dried fruits, such as raisins and apricots, if you like.

Fruit and Yogurt Diet. You can cleanse your colon by eating only fruit, fruit juices, and plain yogurt for one to two days. You may want to do this one day a week. However, if this diet makes you feel weak or very hungry, try adding the Bran-Yo-Lax described below. If this doesn't help, discontinue the diet. Pregnancy is not a time to starve yourself.

Molasses. This is a safe, mild laxative. It can be added to milk or cereal or put on pancakes. One to two tablespoons per day can be used, but discontinue this amount as soon as you achieve the desired result because molasses is also high in calories.

Yogurt or Acidophilus. Either one of these will help stimulate your intestinal bacteria to do a better job of breaking down your food. Eat as much as you like; at least one to two tablespoons of yogurt or one to two teaspoons of acidophilus, one to three times per day.

Bran-Yo-Lax. This recipe combines the laxative properties of yogurt, bran, molasses, and dried fruit. These are minimal amounts. Feel free to use more of any of the ingredients.

Combine 4 tablespoons plain yogurt, 2 tablespoons raw bran, 1 teaspoon molasses, and 1 teaspoon raisins in a bowl.

Eat one to three times a day. At the same time, drink at least one cup of water or juice, which enables the bran to absorb the liquid and expand.

Raw Flaxseed Meal. Many women have obtained relief from this old-time remedy. Just grind the raw flaxseed and add two tablespoons to water, juice, tea, or cereal.

Metamucil. If none of the above remedies are effective, Metamucil is available in drugstores and is safe to use. The main ingredient is psyllium seeds, a natural food substance. Use as directed.

DIARRHEA

Diarrhea is the body's natural process of elimination. It can be a healthy phenomenon if it lasts for just a day or two, but if it goes on for a long time, you will be losing valuable nutrients. The following remedies are safe and effective. If they do not work within a day or two, consult your health care provider.

Apple Sauce. Pectin occurs naturally in apples. It is used in jam making to thicken the syrup, and it does the same for the feces. Apple sauce sprinkled with cinnamon is a painless medicine. Or you can take an apple, peel it (the peel can be difficult to digest), and grate it. There is more pectin in the part of the apple that is closest to the skin.

Acidophilus. Sometimes diarrhea occurs when the intestinal bacteria have been weakened. Lactobacillus acidophilus is a beneficial bacteria which grows naturally in your intestines and elsewhere. Lactobacillus bulgaricus is a similar bacteria which is found in yogurt.

The bacteria count in your intestines can be multiplied by taking acidophilus or eating yogurt. Some forms of yogurt have added acidophilus. Acidophilus is sold in liquid and pill form. Health food stores usually carry both. Most drugstores carry acidophilus tablets. For diarrhea, take one to two tablespoons of the liquid, or one to three tablets, three or four times per day. Some people get good results by eating about four tablespoons (¼ cup) of plain yogurt every two to three hours during their waking hours.

Human mother's milk is a source of acidophilus, so you could make your own yogurt and add 1 tablespoon of mother's milk per cup of milk to start an acidophilus colony growing in it. Mother's milk yogurt is an excellent remedy for chronic digestive disorders.

> **Cinnamon and Cayenne Tea.** This remedy usually takes effect within an hour.
>
> Bring 2 cups of water to a boil and add ¼ teaspoon cinnamon and a dash of cayenne. Simmer for 20 minutes. Cool and strain. Drink a few sips (no more than ¼ cup) every hour.

Bran. Bran is good for diarrhea because it works like a sponge, soaking up excess liquid.

EDEMA

Edema is water retention, characterized by swelling of the feet and ankles. Edema in the last six weeks of pregnancy is a common phenomenon, and there is no need to worry about it if there is proper nourishment and if there is no toxemia. Elevating the feet and hands above the level of the heart relieves swelling by gravity. You can do this several times a day, for ten to fifteen minutes each time. Try to avoid lying on your back because the uterus presses on the large vein, the vena cava, and restricts the blood flow from the legs. Lying on the left side gives the best blood return.

Edema is one symptom in a dangerous syndrome known as toxemia. The other symptoms of toxemia are a significant rise in the blood pressure and protein in the urine. For more information about toxemia, see the index.

Edema is often treated by limiting salt intake, but this practice is changing. It is known now that large amounts of progesterone are secreted during pregnancy, and this hormone increases the amount of sodium (salt) that is excreted from the kidneys. Therefore, salt intake habits need not be changed. Dr. Tom Brewer advises pregnant women to follow high nutrition diets during pregnancy, and he counsels women to salt their food to taste. He has had no cases of toxemia. Sea salt, which is sold in most health food stores, is beneficial to use because it's a good source of important minerals.

Diuretics should not be taken, including herbal diuretics and natural diuretics such as beer and coffee. Diuretics drain the fluid in the blood vessels, which depletes the flow of blood to the baby, diminishing its supply of oxygen and other vital nutrients. So, while a woman may be losing weight, the baby is actually in greater danger.

Vitamin B6 (Pyridoxine). This vitamin is very effective in preventing and eliminating water retention. The usual dosage is 25 to 50 mg. per day. For best results, it should be taken as part of the whole B complex.

FEET: TIRED, SORE, SWOLLEN

It's wonderfully soothing to soak your feet. During pregnancy, you're more likely to suffer from tired, swollen feet because you're carrying excess weight. During the last trimester, natural edema may lead to swollen feet. A foot bath is one of the nicest things you can do for yourself. It refreshes your whole body.

Begin by finding a basin or pot big enough to put in one or both feet, preferably up to the ankle. Then fill the basin with water. Pour this amount of water into a big pot and bring it to a boil. Prepare Epsom salts or comfrey as directed below. When the preparation is ready, fill the basin about one quarter full of cold water, then add some of the hot preparation. Keep the rest in a covered pot so it will stay hot. When the liquid in the basin is comfortably hot, put your feet in. Whenever it begins to cool, add more of the hot preparation.

Epsom Salts. This is a form of magnesium, and it's very soothing. Epsom salts are available in drugstores. Boil two cups of water and add one-half cup of Epsom salts. Use in your foot bath as directed above. Alternately, you can add Epsom salts to your bath water. Boil four cups of water and add one to two cups of Epsom salts. Stir until dissolved and add to your bath.

Comfrey Foot Bath. Boil two cups of water and add two to three handfuls of chopped fresh comfrey leaves, or one to two handfuls of dried crumpled comfrey leaves and simmer for ten minutes. Strain. Add to your foot bath as directed above.

GAS AND HEARTBURN

During pregnancy, your intestines are being squeezed by the growing fetus. Also the increased production of progesterone relaxes your smooth muscles, including your uterus, blood vessels, intestines, stomach, and cardiac sphincter, causing them to become quite lax. Progesterone slows down the peristalsis (contractions) of your intestines and stomach so that food remains longer in the stomach, where it tends to ferment and produce gas. The cardiac sphincter above the stomach is overly relaxed, and the highly acid gastric contents of the stomach then regurgitate into the lower end of the esophagus, eventually causing the inflammation and pain of heartburn. So heartburn doesn't actually involve the heart — it just occurs in the vicinity of the heart, at the bottom of the esophagus, which is just above the stomach.

Do not take baking soda, which upsets the acid-base balance and can be harmful to your developing baby. The same remedies are used for both gas and heartburn.

Yogurt. Eat one to three cups per day. Here's a good recipe for yogurt. It works best with raw milk, when you remove most of the cream. It is excellent with goat's milk.

Slippery Elm. This herb is usually taken in powdered form, in 00 capsules. These are empty gelatin capsules, which are available in most drugstores and health food stores. They hold ¼ teaspoon each, and two caps can be taken, one to three times a day. For best results, swallow the capsule with warm water or tea, which will help it to dissolve. (This is one exception to the advice given earlier to avoid anything that doesn't agreeably pass the intuitive censors of the nose and mouth. In this case, the 00 caps are not used to mask the taste or the smell, but simply to avoid the strange mucilaginous texture of the tea, which most people dislike.)

Slippery Elm Tea. Bring 1 cup of water to a boil and sprinkle in ½ teaspoon of powdered bark, or 1 teaspoon of granulated or plain bark, and simmer for 20 minutes. Strain.

Drink one to three cups per day. Slippery elm is also mildly laxative, tending to make the stools somewhat slippery.

Homemade Yogurt. Put 2 quarts of milk in a pot and cover. Allow the milk to heat gradually until it reaches 180 degrees F. If you don't have a liquid thermometer, just observe the milk periodically. A skin will form on top of the milk, which will increase until an occasional bubble can be seen just beneath the surface of the skin. Eventually the bubbles will gather force and escape to the outer edge. (If you are using goat's milk, this is the time to remove it from the heat.) Allow another minute for more tiny bubbles to form, but do not allow the milk to reach a rolling boil.

Remove the cover and place the pot of hot milk in a basin of cold water, or simply allow it to cool to 98 degrees F. If you don't have a thermometer, you can test it by putting a clean finger into the milk: It should be just barely comfortable to leave your finger in the milk.

Choose a suitable container that will keep the milk at a constant temperature for 6 to 12 hours, until it sets. I use a Yogo-Therm, which has an inner container that holds ½ gallon of milk, and it's surrounded by an outer container that's insulated. There are various yogurt-makers available at health food stores.

Rinse the container with hot water. Then add ¼ cup of plain yogurt for each quart of milk. Add an equal amount of warm milk to the container and stir with a whip. Then add about 1 cup more of warm milk and stir again. Add all of the remaining milk and stir again.

Cover the container and allow to sit for 4 to 8 hours, until it sets. Don't be discouraged if your first attempts don't set; drinking liquid yogurt is just as beneficial for overcoming gas as eating firm yogurt.

HEADACHES

Headaches are common during pregnancy due to hormonal changes.

Calcium. Calcium is good for pain. When taken alone, it tends to quiet your nerves and ease your pain. But if you want a more stimulating effect, take 100 mg. of vitamin C with each dose of calcium. Usually calcium comes

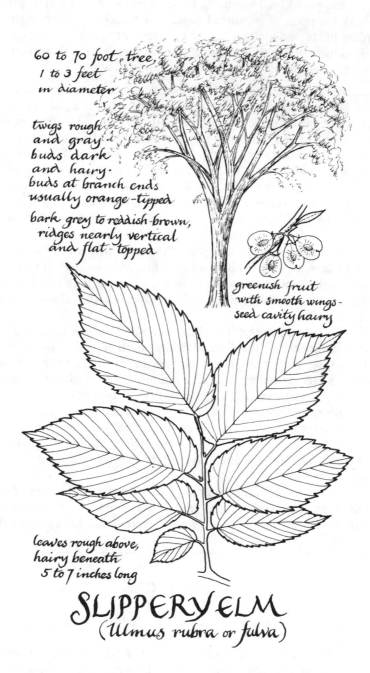

60 to 70 foot tree,
1 to 3 feet
in diameter

twigs rough
and gray
buds dark
and hairy.
buds at branch ends
usually orange-tipped

bark grey to reddish-brown,
ridges nearly vertical
and flat-topped

greenish fruit
with smooth wings-
seed cavity hairy

leaves rough above,
hairy beneath
5 to 7 inches long

SLIPPERY ELM
(Ulmus rubra or fulva)

in tablets of about 450 mg. You may need to take one to four tablets, one to four times per day, depending on how serious the pain is.

Note: If headaches get worse and more frequent, or if they are worse at the upper back of your head, there is a possibility of high blood pressure. If you have a fever of 102 degrees or more along with a headache, with no other symptoms, this could also be dangerous. Consult your health care provider.

Hops, Scullcap, and Catnip. These herbs can be taken as a tea or in capsules for safe and effective relief.

> **Hops, Scullcap, and Catnip.** Bring 2 cups of water to a boil. Remove from the heat. Add 1 teaspoon of each herb. Brew for 20 minutes.
>
> Reheat if desired, but do not boil. Drink one to two cups, as needed. Store the unused portion in the refrigerator.

To take these herbs as capsules, put equal parts of each herb in a seed or coffee grinder or blender and powder them. Then fill empty 00 gelatin capsules with the powdered herbs. Three capsules are equivalent to one cup of tea.

Note: Any one of these herbs, used alone, is also effective for tension headaches.

Acupressure Massage. This works for almost every frontal headache. Ask a friend to proceed as follows: Begin by gently and then firmly rubbing the neck and shoulders. When they feel fairly loose, place your thumb and the third finger of one hand at the base of the skull. With the other hand on her forehead, begin to slowly and gently rub in a circular motion at the points at the base of the skull. Build up to firm pressure, but never to the point of causing pain. Do this for three minutes, then ease off gradually.

Peppermint Oil. Rub peppermint oil into your temples. Most people experience a remarkable easing of tension. Peppermint oil is available in most drugstores. Some people use Essential Balm (described under "Insect Repellents") which contains peppermint oil. You can also drink peppermint tea, or combine it with catnip, scullcap, and/or hops (see recipe above). Peppermint as a tea is good for settling the stomach, which may be the cause of the headache.

HEMORRHOIDS

The rectum is the bottom six to eight inches of the large intestines, and the anus is the last inch of the rectum. The rectum is lined with a mucus membrane and blood vessels run just under this membrane, forming a network of veins around the anus. During pregnancy, the high level of progesterone in your body causes the smooth muscles to relax. The middle layer of the blood vessels consists of smooth muscles. When these muscles relax, it can cause bulging. So pregnancy predisposes a woman to develop varicose veins.

Hemorrhoids are varicose veins occurring around the anus, and they can cause pain, itching, or discomfort in the anal area. You may also notice blood on the stools, or on the toilet paper after wiping. (If the blood is actually mixed with the stools, contact a medical worker.)

When there is pressure on the veins, they swell up. This may be caused by constipation or by the natural enlargement of the uterus during pregnancy. Hemorrhoids may occur inside the rectum, or they may protrude outside the anus. Fatigue and tension make it difficult for the anal sphincter to relax, which can also cause hemorrhoids. Straining to evacuate small, hard feces is a major cause of hemorrhoids, because it causes the veins to fill with blood. Most women have large hemorrhoids during labor due to the pressure of the uterus on the vena cava. With the help of exercise, these disappear soon after giving birth.

Kegel Exercises. These involve developing control over the sphincter muscle, with its openings at the urethra, the vagina, and the anus. You can learn to use this muscle to relax, hold back, or push at any of these openings. The Kegel exercises, which are described in chapter 2 (see index), are directed at gaining control over your vagina, but these same exercises can be directed to your anus, which will help pump the blood out of the enlarged pelvic veins.

Cleanliness. Keeping the anal canal clean is extremely important in treating hemorrhoids. A cotton swab dipped in water can be inserted into your anus to the depth of the cotton. Bearing down makes insertion easier. Repeat this action, using fresh cotton swabs, until they come out clean. Do this after each bowel movement. Then apply witch hazel (available in any drugstore), lemon juice, or vitamin E with a cotton swab. There may be some initial stinging with the first two, but this is a good sign that the hemorrhoids are shrinking.

Vitamin B6. A deficiency of this vitamin can cause hemorrhoids. Take at least 10 mg. per day.

INSECT BITES AND REPELLENTS

Remedies for Bites

These are the most popular natural remedies for bug bites, including mosquitoes, deer flies, and no-see-ums.

Plantain. This weed can be found on practically every unsprayed city lawn and country field. There are two varieties: *Plantago lanceolata* (narrow leaved) and *Plantago major* (broad leaved). Both are equally effective.

Just macerate a fresh leaf and apply it to the bite. This can be done with a mortar and pestle, but most people don't carry these in their pockets, so the easiest way is to wash and then chew it until it's a gob of macerated plantain mixed with saliva. This combines the drawing power of plantain with the healing and soothing properties of saliva. Chewing the plantain helps to release its juices, and when it's mixed with saliva, it will stick to the skin and remain there for a couple of minutes, until it starts to dry, and then it will fall off. This is usually long enough to draw out the poison and remove the pain of the sting.

Plantain is effective for most insect bites, including bee stings. But if you are stung by a bee, take 2,000 to 3,000 mg. of vitamin C, followed by 1,000 mg. per hour, until all symptoms subside. Vitamin C is a natural antihistamine.

Witch Hazel. This is a common drugstore remedy that looks just like alcohol. It's prepared by macerating twigs of witch hazel in water, then it is distilled and about 15 percent ethyl alcohol is added. If you dab a bit of witch hazel on an insect bite, it will relieve the pain and itching immediately. You can dip a cotton swab in the bottle, or just put a little on your finger and apply directly to the bite.

Basic H. This is a liquid soap made by Shaklee Products. According to the sales representative, it is made entirely from vegetable juices. It will take the sting out of your bites when applied full strength. It is also effective as an insect repellent: Just dab it on full strength. Keep it out of your eyes. Incidentally, it's also a good dishwashing detergent, so it's perfect for a camping trip.

Shaklee sales representatives can be found under Health Food Products in the yellow pages.

Insect Repellents

The best cure for insect bites is prevention. But, most commercial insect repellents are made with harmful chemicals, which can be dangerous for your growing baby. There are natural insect repellents that are reasonably good substitutes.

Essential Balm. This is a wonderful ointment, made in China. It contains all natural ingredients: menthol, camphor, peppermint oil, eucalyptus oil, clove oil, cinnamon oil, white camphor oil, and hard and soft paraffin. The odor is pleasant, but it's strong, and most bugs don't like it. The effect lasts about an hour, then begins to fade. Dab it on your hair, forehead, temples, chin, neck, backs of hands, and ankles. It gives a warm sensation, so avoid using on other parts of your face or on mucus membranes. The fumes may irritate the eyes if you use it on your cheeks. I apply it with the little finger of my left hand because then I'm less likely to accidentally put that finger in my eyes or mouth. The balm also helps to relieve itching when bites do occur. It's found in some stores where Chinese items are sold, and some herb and health food stores.

Tiger Balm. This ointment is similar to Essential Balm, and can be used the same way. (Tiger Balm is desribed in more detail under "Aches and Pains.")

Oil of Citronella. Just dab on a few drops of this oil, and most insects will stay away. It smells like mothballs so everyone else might stay away also. But if the bugs are really bad, this is the most effective insect repellent.

LEG CRAMPS

Sudden leg cramps often occur during pregnancy. To stop a cramp when it's occurring, pull the toes and ball of the foot up toward the kneecap (flex the foot).

To prevent further attacks, take up to 1,000 mg. of calcium and 500 mg. of magnesium per day.

Note: If the calf is constantly painful, see a medical worker to find out if phlebitis (vein inflammation) might be the cause.

MORNING SICKNESS, NAUSEA, VOMITING

Nausea occurs most frequently on an empty stomach. Pregnant women are advised to eat about six small meals per day rather than three large ones, both because the stomach capacity becomes smaller as the baby grows larger, and because this keeps the stomach from being empty. Morning sickness also occurs when the blood sugar is low. Honey will give your blood sugar a quick boost, but you'll need some form of protein to keep it high.

Keeping a thermos by the bed with warm milk and honey or molasses works nicely. Many women keep a few crackers by their bedside (preferably whole grain) and eat these on awakening. To avoid feeling dizzy, eat something after you awake and then wait about fifteen minutes before getting out of bed.

Nausea is very common in early pregnancy, but if it persists, there may be underlying fears which need to be worked through. Spend some time alone, or with a friend you really trust, and air out all your fears, no matter how foolish they seem.

Research shows that stress contributes to morning sickness, so do whatever you can to minimize sources of stress in your life.

If the problem persists to the point of weight loss, be sure to consult your doctor or midwife.

The following remedies can be used separately or in combination with each other.

Ginger. This is an effective remedy for the nausea of morning sickness and it's also used for motion sickness. Ginger capsules are available in some health food stores. If you can't find them, powdered ginger can be put into 00 gelatin capsules (both are available in health food stores and powdered ginger also can be purchased in supermarkets). For motion sickness, take two or three capsules half an hour before the expected motion. Follow with half a cup of warm water. For morning sickness, take three or four capsules on arising each day, followed by half a cup of warm water or milk. Wait at least five minutes before getting out of bed. Whenever you feel queasy during the day, take three or four more capsules. Alternately, you can prepare ginger tea and drink one or two cups in the morning or whenever you feel nauseated. It's delicious with milk and honey.

> **Ginger Tea**. Boil 4 cups of water and add 2 tablespoons of fresh grated ginger. Simmer for 20 minutes.

Vitamin B6 (Pyridoxine). Take 10 to 20 mg. of vitamin B6 one to three times per day, as needed, according to the severity of the problem. B6 should be taken as part of the B complex.

Raspberry Leaf, Peppermint, and Peach Leaf Tea. Any of these herbs taken separately or in any combination is also effective. Drink three cups per day.

> **Raspberry Leaf, Peppermint, and Peach Leaf Tea**. Boil 1 cup of water and pour over 1 teaspoon of raspberry leaf, peppermint, and peach leaf. Steep in a covered nonaluminum pot for 5 minutes.

NERVOUS TENSION

It's important to get daily exercise (preferably outdoors), adequate sleep so that you're not exhausted when you wake up, a good diet, and some pleasure in your life. If you aren't getting these things, then don't expect miracles from any of these remedies. If you live under conditions of constant stress, you may want to reevaluate your life-style.

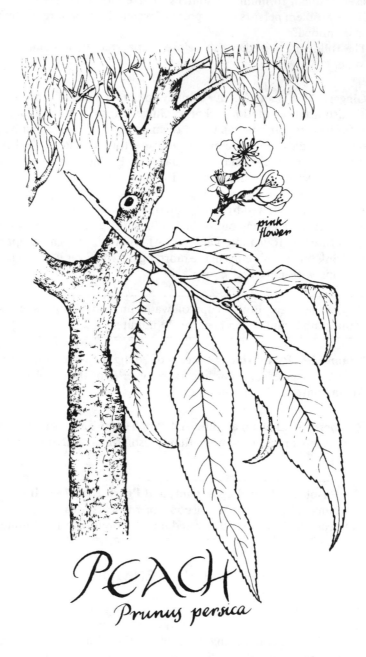

pink flower

PEACH
Prunus persica

Nervous tension often develops as a result of personal problems. Until the cause of tension is discovered and overcome, any remedy will only be temporary. If something is seriously bothering you, find a friend or a therapist you can trust. When grief or anger are repressed, they come out as sickness and tension in your body.

The food you eat feeds your nerves. Refined foods (white sugar and white flour) are "empty"—the essential vitamins and minerals have been removed. Yet these foods require B vitamins for their assimilation, so they'll rob your body of its store of B vitamins for their own digestion. A lack of B1 causes nervous irritability, insomnia, poor memory, and vague fears. A lack of B2 causes degeneration of nervous tissues and mental confusion. A lack of B3 causes mental depression, irritability, fatigue headaches, aches and pains, and loss of memory.

The following remedies will help you to feel better.

Herbs

Many herbs can be taken to strengthen and feed the nerves while easing nervous irritability and pain. They may be used separately or in combination.

Hops. Beer is made with hops, which is one reason why beer can be calming. Hops are excellent for nervous tension. Drink one cup of hops tea hot, morning and evening.

> **Hops Tea**. Boil 1½ cups water. Add 1 teaspoon hops and simmer for 10 minutes.

Scullcap. This herb is soothing to the nerves. It's also helpful for relieving sexual tension.

> **Scullcap Tea**. Bring 1 cup water to a boil. Put 1 teaspoon scullcap in a teapot and add water. Brew for 5 minutes.

Catnip. This gentle herb is very calming. It's good for children and for preventing nightmares.

> **Catnip Tea**. Put 1 teaspoon catnip in a teapot and add 1 cup boiling water. Brew for 3 to 5 minutes.

Hops, Scullcap, and Catnip. You can make a tea of all three herbs. Drink one to two cups, as needed. Store the unused portion in the refrigerator.

> **Hops, Scullcap, and Catnip Tea**. Bring 2 cups water to a boil. Remove from the heat. Add 1 teaspoon of each herb. Brew for 20 minutes. Reheat if desired, but do not boil.

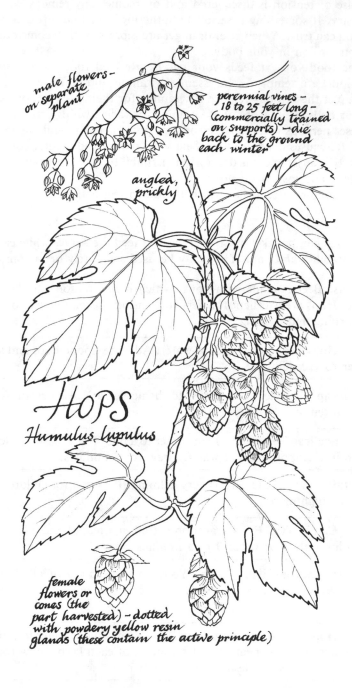

male flowers—
on separate
plant

perennial vines—
18 to 25 feet long—
(commercially trained
on supports)—die
back to the ground
each winter

angled,
prickly

HOPS
Humulus lupulus

female
flowers or
cones (the
part harvested)—dotted
with powdery yellow resin
glands (these contain the active principle)

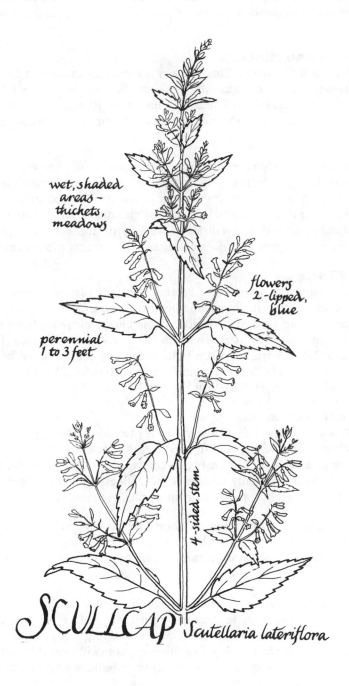

wet, shaded
areas –
thickets,
meadows

flowers
2-lipped,
blue

perennial
1 to 3 feet

4-sided stem

SCULLCAP *Scutellaria lateriflora*

Another way to take these herbs is to put equal parts of each herb in a seed or coffee grinder or blender and powder them. Then fill empty 00 gelatin capsules with the powdered herbs. Three capsules are equivalent to one cup of this tea.

Vitamins and Minerals

Vitamin B Complex. This vitamin is especially important for a healthy nervous system. The dosage will vary according to the severity of your tension, but an average dose would contain about 10 mg. of B2, B3, and B6, taken three times a day. Or take a tablet that contains 25 to 50 mg. once a day.

Calcium and Magnesium. Calcium relaxes the nerves, eases pain, relieves nervous headaches and muscle tension, and encourages sleep. When taken alone, it tends to be very relaxing, but if you need to stay alert and energetic, take it with at least 100 mg. of vitamin C. Magnesium maintains the normal functions of the brain, spinal cord, and nerves. Magnesium is necessary for assimilation of calcium, so supplements often contain both.

Calms Forte

This is a homeopathic preparation that contains plant extracts of passion flower, chamomile, oats, hops, and biochemic phosphates of lime, iron, potash, magnesia, and sodium chloride. These biochemic phosphates (cell salts) are in a form that permits ready assimilation and diffusion into the cells of the body. Calms Forte are little tablets that are sold in some health food stores, or they can be ordered from Standard Homeopathic Company, P.O. Box 61067, Los Angeles, California 90061.

External Treatments

Massage. This is a favorite remedy for tension. When the healing power of touch combines with a skillful massage, the benefits are immeasurable. A good massage on a regular basis prevents your body from building up tensions that could eventually lead to chronic illness. Massage should never be harsh or extremely intense or painful during pregnancy.

Yoga and Deep Breathing. A good exercise (asana) for the whole body is the Salutation to the Sun. Alternate nostril breathing has a very calming effect. *Prenatal Yoga and Natural Birth* by Jeannine Parvatti describes asanas that are beneficial to use during pregnancy.

Herbal Bath. A sweet-smelling bath is a wonderful way to alleviate aches and pains, muscle cramps, tension, and even insomnia and headaches — it soothes away every tense spot in your body. If you remain in the bath for more than twenty-five minutes, you will probably fall asleep in the tub. For a recipe of herbs to add to your bath, see "Aches and Pains."

Insomnia

The following remedies should help you to sleep. But if you can't get to sleep, it's probably better to get up and do something you want to do instead of just lying there feeling frustrated.

Hops, Catnip, and Scullcap Tea. Prepare as directed under "Headaches." One cup of this tea will help you to relax, and two to three cups will make you feel sleepy.

Herbal Bath. Prepare as described above. It will help you to relax and may make you feel quite sleepy if you stay in for over twenty-five minutes.

Sleepy-Time Tea. This pleasant-tasting herb tea is made by Celestial Seasonings and is available in most health food stores. Many people enjoy having a cup or two just before bed and find that it helps them to sleep better. It contains chamomile, spearmint, tilia, passion flowers, lemon grass, raspberry leaves, orange blossoms, hawthorn berries, scullcap, rosebuds, and hops.

Calcium. A lack of calcium results in insomnia. Many people like to drink a cup of hot milk with honey or molasses just before bedtime to calm their nerves. Honey and molasses are concentrated sources of calcium, and honey raises the level of calcium in the blood. Milk is high in calcium and neutralizes stomach acid. It also contains tryptophan, an amino acid that helps to induce sleep. See the index for more sources of calcium.

Hops Pillow. The soothing smell of the hops will help you to relax and fall asleep. Use a generous amount of dried hops and sprinkle with a little alcohol to activate its properties. You can make a small pillow, and tuck it inside the pillowcase along with your regular pillow.

Depression and Paranoia

The usual treatment for this common condition is anti-depressant drugs. But particularly during pregnancy, you want to avoid using such drugs, because it has been shown that they may contribute to causing Down's Syndrome and other problems for your unborn child.

Instead of using drugs, consider taking a nutritional approach to your mental health. Begin by eliminating refined foods such as white sugar and white flour, which rob your body of B vitamins. One of these vitamins is B3 (niacin). A lack of this nutrient upsets the higher brain centers, causing mental depression, irritability, loss of sense of humor, loss of memory, hallucinations, difficulty sleeping, and fatigue. Large doses of this vitamin have resulted in dramatic improvement in cases of paranoia and even schizophrenia. An average dose is 25 to 100 mg. of niacin per day, taken as part of the B complex.

SPOTTING, THREATENED MISCARRIAGE

Be sure to notify your doctor or midwife if spotting occurs. Miscarriage is an all too common occurrence. About one out of every four conceptions does not result in a live birth. The first things to consider are: 1) Do you have a good diet? A pregnant woman's diet should be very nutritious. If you can't stomach much food, then take plenty of vitamin and mineral supplements. 2) Is this really a good time for you to have a baby? If not, it may be better to let go of this baby and wait until the circumstances are more favorable. Sometimes the body has its own wisdom. Don't cling to a baby your body rejects; the child could be brain-damaged or otherwise impaired.

If you're quite sure you want the baby now and that the time and the circumstances are appropriate, here are some procedures to help avoid a miscarriage. All of the following may be used together.

Bed Rest. Go to bed. Elevate your feet to a level above your abdomen. Get plenty of rest until the spotting stops entirely.

Vitamin E (Alpha Tocopherols). Take 400 I.U. per day of natural vitamin E (preferably), or 800 I.U. of synthetic vitamin E. Be sure to get alpha tocopherols because they're more effective than mixed tocopherols in preventing miscarriages. After the spotting stops, reduce to 200 I.U. daily of natural or 400 I.U. of synthetic vitamin E. Continue this amount for another two to four weeks. Avoid all refined foods and eat only whole grain products, which are naturally high in vitamin E.

Note: The word "tocopherol" means childbearing. Vitamin E will also enable the child to make better use of oxygen, thereby reducing the danger of brain damage and other birth defects.

> **Raspberry Leaf Tea**. Drink two or three cups per day. Pour 1 cup o3f boiling water over 1 teaspoon raspberry leaves. Add 1 teaspoon peppermint or any other tea you like for flavor. Steep in a covered pot for 5 minutes. Strain and drink. Add honey if desired.

Black Haw. This herb is a uterine sedative. Take a half cup of black haw tea, twice a day. If your flow increases, take three to four times a day. When the flow ceases, continue to take one cup daily for one week, then one cup every other day for one week. Do not take more than the stated amount because an overdose may lower your blood pressure. If your blood pressure is already low, don't use this herb. If black haw is unavailable, or if your blood pressure is low, you can substitute cramp bark.

> **Black Haw Tea**. Cover 1 teaspoon of the powdered bark with 1 cup boiling water and steep in covered pot for 15 minutes. Or simmer 2 teaspoons bark in 1¼ cups of water for 20 minutes (about ¼ cup will evaporate).

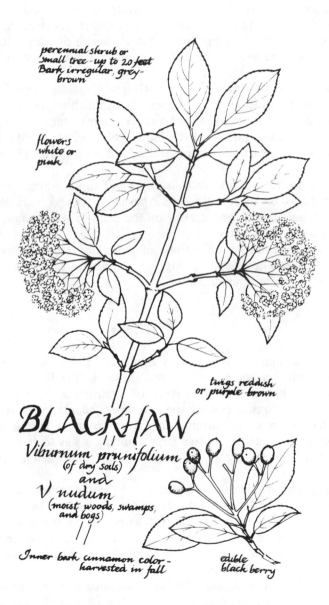

perennial shrub or
small tree - up to 20 feet
Bark irregular, grey-
brown

flowers
white or
pink

twigs reddish
or purple brown

BLACKHAW

Viburnum prunifolium
(of dry soils)
and
V nudum
(moist woods, swamps,
and bogs)

Inner bark cinnamon color -
harvested in fall

edible
black berry

STOMACH OR INTESTINAL FLU

The flu is caused by a virus in the digestive system. It's characterized by nausea, vomiting, diarrhea, cramps, and loss of interest in food. There may be headaches and fever. It usually goes away by itself within twenty-four to forty-eight hours. If the symptoms are very severe, consider the possibility of dysentery or food poisoning, and consult a health care provider. Prevention of the flu is the same as for colds (check under "Cold Prevention" for details).

Slippery Elm, Cinnamon, and Ginger Capsules. This is an effective herbal remedy, which usually takes effect within about ten minutes. To make the capsules, combine 1 tablespoon slippery elm, 1 tablespoon ginger, and 1 teaspoon cinnamon powders. Mix thoroughly. Fill empty 00 gelatin capsules (available in most drugstores and health food stores), which hold ¼ teaspoon each.

Take one to two caps, followed by a half cup of warm water, up to four times per day, for up to four days. Alternately, put ¼ teaspoon of the mixture on a butter knife and drop it on the back of your tongue and swallow quickly with warm water.

It's a good idea to have some of these stomach capsules already prepared, because when you're feeling sick and nauseated you may not have the patience to prepare them.

STRESS

Stress is a normal part of life. Any significant change will produce stress in the body, whether it's the severe stress caused by the death of a close family member, or the relatively mild stress of a Christmas holiday.

We have two choices when meeting stress: adaptation or resistance. I believe that the most important adaptation to stress is emotional release. Whenever we are under unusual stress, finding a way to express our feelings helps to alleviate the pressure. Stress is normal, but when it builds up, it becomes distress.

Pregnancy produces a dramatic change in our bodies and in our concept of ourselves. If we anticipate this change with pleasure, we can usually adapt to it without much difficulty. But if it is unexpected, if the circumstances are difficult, and if we resist the change, we are more likely to see the effects of stress turning into distress, and taking a toll on our health (and indirectly on our baby's mental and physical health).

One of the most serious illnesses associated with pregnancy is toxemia, and doctors still haven't found the cause. It is characterized by protein in the urine, edema, high blood pressure, and rapid weight gain—all characteristics of severe stress.

Stress and illness are characterized by the following syndrome:

1. Proteins are drawn from the thymus and lymph glands and broken down to form blood sugar for energy. If the stress continues for a long time, these glands shrink, fewer white blood cells are produced, and the body's self-defense system is weakened.

2. Blood pressure increases.

3. Minerals are drawn from the bones. This explains why you get an aching feeling in your bones when you're sick.

4. Fat is mobilized from fatty tissues, which is why continued stress can cause peptic ulcers.

5. Salt is retained. People who are under continuous stress tend to look puffy, especially in the face. There is often edema and weight gain.

If your diet is good, you can experience periods of stress without harm. But during periods of extreme stress (distress), you will need to supplement your diet in order to avoid nervousness and illness. The following are the essential nutrients you will need while under significant stress.

Vitamin B Complex. A balanced B vitamin complex will provide vitamin B2, pantothenic acid, and choline, which are essential for the production of natural cortisone in the body. The adrenal cortex also requires B2 and pantothenic acid. The dosage will vary according to the severity of the stress, but an average dose for a person under significant stress is a tablet that contains about 10 mg. of B2, B3, and B6 three times a day, or a tablet that contains 25 to 50 mg. taken once a day.

Vitamin C. This vitamin is essential to the functioning of the adrenal cortex. During times of severe stress, be sure to take at least 250 mg., three times a day. Ascorbic acid is less expensive than the natural forms of vitamin C, and it is adequate for treating stress.

Vitamin E. This vitamin is more concentrated in the pituitary gland than in any other part of the body. It prevents the pituitary and adrenal hormones from being destroyed by oxygen. An average dose for times of stress is about 400 I.U. once a day. (If you have had high blood pressure or rheumatic heart disease, begin with 100 I.U. and increase by 100 units every six weeks.)

Vitamin A. This vitamin is important for the optimum functioning of the adrenal cortex. A healthy dose is a 10,000 I.U. per day.

Whenever I'm under stress, I take supplements of vitamins B and C. If the stress increases, I also take vitamins A and E. The latter are oil soluble and should be taken with milk or with a meal, or some source of fat.

STRETCH MARKS AND ITCHING

During pregnancy, as your body expands, it sometimes leaves stretch marks, particularly on the belly and breasts. To avoid or minimize stretch marks (and the itching that often accompanies them), rub vitamin E oil or cream or coconut oil or olive oil into your breasts and abdomen daily during your pregnancy.

After your baby is born, if you have stretch marks, try vitamin E. Use 400 I.U. capsules, and puncture them with a pin to squeeze out the oil onto the stretch marks. Also take 200 to 800 I.U. orally per day. There is a wide range of responsiveness to this treatment. Some women have excellent results and others are not helped at all.

TOXEMIA

This is a syndrome or combination of symptoms which include edema, protein in the urine, and a significant rise above normal blood pressure (a rise of 30 mm. of mercury, systolic, and 15 mm. diastolic). The term toxemia is misleading, because there are no toxins in the blood. In fact, the cause of this disease is still unknown, though the symptoms are all characteristic of stress.

The early stage of this disease is called preeclampsia, and if it begins early in pregnancy, it can cause malformations; if it begins later, it can cause low birth weight or death of the baby. The most severe stage, eclampsia, can be fatal for both mother and child. It is rarely seen in North America, where women are carefully monitored throughout pregnancy.

If preeclampsia does occur, concentrate on reducing stress, make sure you are getting *adequate* protein, eliminate foods that contain empty calories, and increase your intake of fresh vegetables and fruits. Preeclampsia tends to occur most commonly among teenagers fifteen years and under and women over forty-five. Statistics show twice as many cases of toxemia among women bearing their first child in their late thirties as compared to those in their twenties. Yet Dr. Tom Brewer cites a study of women of all ages, which compares two groups of 750 women. One group was given a highly nutritious diet, and the control group had a normal diet. The high-nutrition group had no preeclampsia and no eclampsia. The control group had 59 cases of preeclampsia and 5 cases of eclampsia.

Since doctors don't know the cause of toxemia, in the past they just treated the symptoms—with very poor results. This method of treatment or so-called prevention has been abandoned by most physicians. But older mothers may remember being told to restrict their weight gain, cut down on salt, and take diuretics.

It is now known that edema by itself is not an ominous sign. In fact, women with edema have slightly larger babies than those without, and they have fewer premature babies. When women eat nutritious foods, those who are heavier tend to gain more water weight, which comes off easily after the baby is weaned, while those who are thinner gain more fat.

It has been shown that restriction of salt does not prevent toxemia. During pregnancy you have additional fluid in your body, and the kidneys eliminate more sodium. You need to have a balance of sodium in your fluids, so your body requires salt to maintain your health.

As for diuretics, the American College of Obstetrics and Gynecology has stated that diuretics do not prevent toxemia and should not be taken for edema.

Preeclampsia is most commonly a disease of the last trimester, in women who are pregnant for the first time. When it's encountered in the second trimester, it's especially dangerous to the mother and the fetus. Hypertension is difficult to control, and since it may lead to eclampsia, the pregnancy may have to be terminated, or labor induced (amniocentesis may be used to determine the exact age of the baby and its chances for survival).

When edema is accompanied by swelling of the lower limbs, hands, and face, even in the early morning, this could be an early sign of preeclampsia and should be reported to your caregiver immediately. When these symptoms progress to vomiting, frontal headaches, visual disturbances, and very rapid weight gain, this indicates a serious deterioration of your condition.

Long-standing or undetected preeclampsia can cause intra-uterine growth retardation which leads to dangerously low birth weight babies. Preeclampsia interferes with the efficient nourishment of the fetus through the placenta. High blood pressure causes vasospasm—a spasm of the blood vessels—which decreases the oxygen supply to the placenta. During labor, the stress of contractions, together with vasospasm, decreases oxygen available to the fetus. This may necessitate early induction of labor with careful electronic fetal monitoring. If fetal distress develops, a cesarean may be required.

If you have any sign of high blood pressure or toxemia, make sure that you are getting *at least* 800 mcg. of folic acid per day.

TURNING THE BABY

Before the ninth month in utero, most babies are positioned with their head up, but this is not the best position to get born in. Before the last few weeks of pregnancy, nature provides our bodies with a spontaneous impulse to turn the baby. Your doctor or midwife can tell you if your baby has turned.

If your baby is not in an upside-down position two weeks before your due date, there is the probability of a breech birth, which can be difficult, and can make having a home birth somewhat dangerous. There are some midwives and doctors who have the rare skill of being able to turn a baby in utero, with their hands.

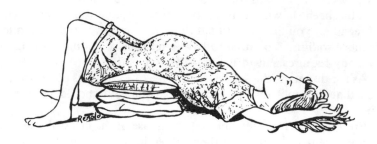

Fortunately there are other ways to achieve the same result.

Pulsatilla. This is a homeopathic remedy which many women have used successfully to turn their babies. They took 12X potency tablets, under the tongue, one per day for up to two weeks. These can be ordered from Standard Homeopathic Company, P.O. Box 61037, Los Angeles, California 90061. Do not attempt to make your own tea with pulsatilla. This is a homeopathic remedy and must be prepared according to homeopathic principles.

Tilt Posture. Place two or three pillows on the floor and sit on them. Then lie with your head on the floor so that your pelvis is raised nine to twelve inches above your head. Do this twice a day on an empty stomach for ten minutes. Begin at the thirtieth week of pregnancy, and continue for four to six weeks or until the baby turns. After it turns do *not* continue the exercise or it may turn back again.

URINATING EXCESSIVELY

Depending on the anatomical relationship between a particular woman's bladder and her uterus, she may have to urinate more frequently. It's normal to urinate a lot during pregnancy—at least once every four hours. As the uterus grows and presses on the bladder, you may urinate more and more frequently—sometimes as often as every hour.

If there is pain during urination, or if the urine appears cloudy (you can urinate into a glass jar to check it), have the urine analyzed to see if there is a bladder infection. If you do have an infection, check under "Bladder Infection" for remedies. Otherwise, the following exercise can be used to strengthen the kidneys, making urination less frequent.

Taoist Exercise. When you wake up in the morning, place your hands on your bare back, just over your kidneys, which are located on either side of your spine above the waist. Rub downwards, thirty-six times, once a day. You should notice a difference within a week, but you must continue to do this exercise daily if you want to maintain the effect. If there is no change within a week, then this exercise probably will not work for you.

VAGINAL INFECTIONS

Normally, glucose (blood sugar) is exuded from the blood serum into the vagina to keep it moist. The friendly organisms that grow in the vagina metabolize the glucose and the by-product is lactic acid. This creates an acidic environment in the vagina. During pregnancy, an increase in pelvic blood supply and an increase in the activity of friendly organisms can produce a clear or whitish discharge which may get heavier during the last month. This discharge is normal during pregnancy.

However, the vast hormonal and chemical changes that occur during pregnancy can cause an overgrowth of these otherwise friendly organisms, which can produce a whitish or yellowish discharge that is smelly, irritating, itchy, and/or curdish. This is probably an infection, and it should be treated. You can begin by trying home remedies for a week or two, especially if you are willing to use garlic (as described below) — since garlic is effective for almost all forms of vaginitis. But if you don't get results within two weeks, be sure to see a medical worker. Gonorrhea could cause these symptoms, and it should be ruled out.

Women with stubborn vaginal infections may have an overgrowth of *candida* (yeast) throughout their system. A naturopath or knowledgeable doctor can determine if you have *candida* and can explain how to treat it with diet, garlic, acidophilus, and possibly antifungal medication. For more information, read *Back to Health* by Dennis Remington, M.D.

Once you know exactly what kind of infection you have, it will be easier to determine which remedies to use. All vaginal infections are hard to get rid of until after the birth, so you may have to be satisfied with just suppressing the symptoms.

General Prevention
Wear cotton underpants, or none at all. Try to avoid leotards and tights made of synthetics which provide the perfect warm, moist environment for the growth of yeast.

Wipe from front to back after a bowel movement. Don't share wash-cloths or towels. Avoid soap, because it's alkaline.

Minimize sugar, sweets, and refined foods because yeast grows on sugar.

Get enough rest so you don't feel tired in the morning. Make sure your diet is adequate in vitamins A, B, and C. Minimize stress.

Avoid commercial douches or frequent douches of any kind which wash away the beneficial natural secretions. Avoid feminine hygiene deodorants. A good substitute is a tablet of acidophilus inserted into the vagina before going to bed at night. These are available in most drugstores and health food stores.

Preventive Cleanliness

Washing the vagina with clear running water can be an effective way to prevent vaginitis. The natural acid secretions provide the perfect chemistry for cleansing and purifying the vagina. Anything that changes this acidic climate makes a woman more vulnerable to infection. This explains why acid substances, like vinegar, are used in the treatment of vaginitis. The opposite of acid is alkaline, so anything that is alkaline is potentially disruptive inside the vagina. This includes semen, menstrual fluid, lochia (the blood flow after childbirth), and soap. Soap should never be used in the vagina. There are some expensive acid soaps, but why pay for what you already have? The natural acidic discharge from the vagina is self-cleansing. A healthy woman only needs to wash regularly with plain water and after each time she has intercourse (it doesn't have to be immediately after—the next morning is adequate). If there is an infection or irritation, a daily wash with a vinegar rinse is advisable.

Vinegar Rinse. Add two teaspoons white vinegar (don't use apple cider vinegar because it may ferment) to one cup of water. Squat in the bathtub or over a large bowl. It's not necessary to remove clothes that can be kept above the waist. You may want to close the drain on the tub and run a little warm water so it won't be cold to your feet. Dip your finger into the vinegar solution and then insert it into your vagina and move it around inside. Then rinse your finger under the tap or in another bowl of fresh water. You may see a white discharge. Repeat this several times, or until the discharge is gone. The whole process only takes a few minutes.

Encourage your partner to wash after intercourse. Uncircumcised men are more likely to be carriers of vaginal infections. This could be indicated by little red spots on the foreskin. Men can also wash with a solution of two teaspoons of white vinegar in one cup of water.

When treating vaginal infections, try to avoid intercourse, which irritates the fragile vaginal tissues and introduces alkaline semen to the area. If you do have intercourse, ask your partner to use a condom and always make sure there is plenty of lubrication. Cocoa oil or vegetable oil makes a good lubricant.

> **Homemade Lubricant**. Make a strong tea by adding 2 tablespoons of slippery elm powder to 1 cup of boiling water. Simmer for 10 minutes. This is an excellent lubricant.

Garlic Suppositories. Prepare a garlic suppository by carefully peeling one small or medium-size clove of garlic. Try not to nick it or it may burn. Dip it in vegetable oil (to prevent burning) and insert it into the vagina like a tampon. It into an be easily removed, like a diaphragm, by inserting your finger behind it and popping it out.

Remove the garlic every twelve hours and insert a fresh clove. Do this for three to five days. Don't be surprised if your discharge increases at first; this is the body's way of cleansing itself before the healing begins. However, if you experience a significant amount of burning or irritation, remove the garlic.

Yeast Infections

Yeast is a fungus that normally grows in the vagina. Overgrowth of yeast in the vagina is characterized by itching, unpleasant odor, irritation, and a whitish discharge that resembles cottage cheese. If you have a yeast infection when you give birth, your baby will probably get yeast in its digestive tract. This is called thrush. Thrush can sometimes be remedied by giving the child one teaspoon of acidophilus three times a day.

Garlic. Use as directed earlier in this section.

Acidophilus. Lactobacillus acidophilus is a bacteria that grows naturally in the vagina. It ferments the vaginal secretions to make them acidic. Yeast also grows normally in the vagina, but when there is an overgrowth of yeast, a yeast infection occurs. Lactobacillus bulgaricus, or yogurt, is another form of the same bacteria.

Acidophilus comes in liquid and tablet form. A rinse can be made with the liquid, using two teaspoons in one cup of water and applying it as with the vinegar rinse described earlier in this section. The easiest method is to use acidophilus tablets. Insert one or two tablets in your vagina each night before going to bed. The infection usually clears up within seven to ten days. Both the liquid and the tablets can be obtained from drugstores and health food stores.

Yogurt. Lactobacillus bulgaricus ferments milk to make yogurt, just as the beneficial bacteria in the vagina ferment vaginal secretions to make them acidic. One to two tablespoons of plain, unsweetened yogurt can be inserted with a vaginal applicator. Or dissolve two tablespoons of yogurt in one cup of warm water and use this as a rinse, applying it as with the vinegar rinse described earlier in this section. Whatever method is used, it should be repeated once a day for a week or twice a week until the infection is gone.

Vinegar Rinse. This remedy, as described earlier in this section, works best when used at the first sign of an infection. Some women like to rinse with vinegar each day and then insert an acidophilus pill each night for one week.

Baking Soda Rinse and Alkaline Diet. Most women get vaginal infections because their vagina is not acidic enough, but some women's vaginas are too acidic. If the above remedies do not work for you, or if they make you worse, try the baking soda rinse and the alkaline diet.

To make the rinse, combine two teaspoons of baking soda with one cup of water and rinse as with the vinegar rinse described earlier in this section. Sometimes it's helpful to eat foods that have an alkaline reaction in the body. Acid and alkaline are confusing terms because in this context we call foods such as citrus fruits alkaline. In fact, this does not refer to the acid content of the food but rather to a process that occurs within the body. Foods combine with oxygen and then are "burned up" by the body, thus leaving a residue or "ash." This residue is then analyzed for its mineral content. If it is highest in sodium, potassium, calcium, and magnesium, it is called alkaline producing. If it is highest in sulfur, phosphorus, chlorine, and uncombusted organic acid radicals, it is called acid producing. Try the following diet for two weeks. If you like the results, you may want to continue it longer.

More than two-thirds of your diet should be alkaline-forming foods. This includes almost all vegetables and fruits. (The exceptions are cranberries and large plums or prunes, which have a slightly acid reaction.) All vegetables, including potatoes and sweet potatoes are alkaline. Also lima beans, dried peas, red beans, soybeans (including soy sauce, miso, tofu, etc.), almonds, chestnuts, honey, sunflower seed oil, and sesame seed oil are alkaline.

The following foods are neutral or nearly neutral and can be eaten freely: blueberries, apples, watermelon, sweet corn, fresh green peas, asparagus, olive oil, filbert nuts, egg yolks, butter, goat's milk, cheese, nonfat raw milk (whole milk is more acidic), and chocolate.

Less than one-third of your diet should be selected from acid-forming foods, such as grains, beans (except those listed above) and lentils, nuts (except those listed above), meat, fish, poultry, sugar, and egg whites.

A sample diet might go as follows. For breakfast: cornmeal mush with milk, or fruit with yogurt, or a vegetable omelet with one piece of toast and butter. Snack: apple. Lunch: vegetable soup with a roll, or a large salad with an open-faced grilled cheese sandwich with mushrooms and alfalfa sprouts. Snack: celery sticks with peanut butter. Dinner: stir-fried rice with vegetables, or baked potato with broccoli and fish or meat, or refried red beans with tortillas and lettuce and tomato and a sprinkling of grated cheese. For beverages, drink one glass each of apple juice, carrot juice, and milk.

Trichomoniasis (Trichomonas)

This infection is caused by a microscopic protozoa with a tail (*Trichomonas vaginalis*). Women who have trichomonas experience a yellow to yellowish-green discharge, itching, burning, and a fishy odor. Symptoms may be worse before and after your period. A trichomonas infection can cause a bladder infection because the protozoa may be moved out of the vaginal opening and up to the urethra during intercourse.

The standard treatment is Flagyl, but Flagyl has caused gene mutations and birth defects and cancer in animals. It should not be used during pregnancy.

Unfortunately, herbal alternatives for trichomonas are among the least impressive home remedies. My survey indicates that none of them are more than 50 percent effective. This is not surprising since only extremely potent medications have been effective in killing off this stubborn protozoa. Nevertheless, since Flagyl is so harmful, it is certainly worth trying a home remedy. *Note*: Your partner(s) must also follow the procedure described for them below.

Garlic Suppository. Use as directed earlier in this section.

Spermicidal Jelly. Researchers in the *British Journal of Venereal Diseases* report that spermicidal jellies (like the kind used with diaphragms) inhibit the growth of trichomoniasis and possibly yeast. Some women who are very susceptible to trichomonas infections (for example, many women who use birth control pills) have found that using spermicidal jelly once every two weeks can prevent trich. This is not a natural organic remedy, but the chemicals in spermicides are relatively harmless. During an infection, the spermicide can be inserted with a foam applicator before you go to sleep each night for five to seven days. Do this after you get into bed because the warmth of your body will cause the spermicide to melt, and it will just drip out if you get up. Both the jelly and the applicator are available in drugstores. *Note*: If you find one brand of spermicide irritating, try another brand. For some women, spermicide seems to aggravate a trichomonas infection.

Treatments for Men

Men are carriers of trichomonas, and it can be passed during sexual intercourse, even though men are usually asymptomatic. Men *must* be treated. If you want to avoid Flagyl, the treatment is to not ejaculate for ten days. Apparently the protozoa are nourished by semen. But there are some stubborn cases where the trichomonads survive in the prostate and seminal vesicles, so be sure to get checked by a medical worker after ten days to be certain you've gotten rid of the organism. It is also advisable to get plenty of rest, a good diet, and to eat one clove of raw garlic a day.

Hemophilus

The symptoms of *Hemophilus vaginalis* are similar to those of trichomonas, although the discharge may be creamy white or grayish and particularly foul-smelling after intercourse. It is transmitted primarily through sexual intercourse, so your partner must be treated also. The treatment for men is the same as for trichomonas, as described above.

Garlic and Vinegar. Alternate the garlic suppository (described earlier in this section) with the vinegar rinse (described earlier in this section) from night to night for one to two weeks, until the symptoms disappear. Some individuals have had good results with garlic suppositories alone for five days.

Nonspecific Vaginitis

This is a term used for vaginal infections other than yeast, trichomonas, and *Hemophilus*. Nonspecific vaginitis may be characterized by a white or yellow or possibly bloody discharge. There may be lower back pain, cramps, and swollen glands in the abdomen and inner thighs. The treatment is to use garlic suppositories as described earlier in this section. *Note*: Men are not always treated, but if the garlic suppositories do not work for you, ask your partner to try the treatment described for trichomonas, and after five days, repeat the garlic treatment.

VARICOSE VEINS

The increased production of progesterone during pregnancy will cause the veins throughout your body to become lax. This relaxes your uterus, which prevents spontaneous abortion. But it also makes the walls of your arteries and veins less resilient. When the growing uterus puts pressure up against your pelvic veins, it causes them to become engorged and bulge into varicose veins.

Walking and exercising provide the best prevention. The veins flow through your muscles and during exercise the muscles contract, which assists blood return. Elevation of your legs is beneficial in collapsing the veins, giving them a rest. Likewise, placing your chest lower than your hips by getting down on your elbows and knees brings your uterus up and out of the pelvis, allowing better drainage for the veins of your legs. A daily dose of at least 100 mg. of vitamin C will help to keep your veins healthy and elastic.

After your twenty-sixth week, try to avoid lying on your back, because the uterus presses on the large vein, the vena cava, restricting blood flow to your legs. Lying on your left side gives the best blood return.

Most ailments have emotional as well as physical causes. The underlying cause for varicose veins tends to be a secret desire to kick somebody. Vigorously kicking a pillow relieves tension and gives the legs exercise at the same time. This can be quite effective. Try using a big pillow, and put it up against the wall in a corner of the room.

Most women have been well-trained to hold in their anger and be "nice." This is not a bad idea when it comes to public relations, but it puts stress on your body to hold in a lot of anger and resentment. If you can give yourself permission to release your emotions in the privacy of your own room, you won't harm anyone, and you will probably feel a lot better.

Vitamin E. This vitamin helps to eliminate varicose veins. Take 400 to 800 I.U. per day. (If you've had rheumatic heart disease or high blood pressure, begin with 100 I.U. and increase by 100 units every six weeks.)

REFERENCES

Herman Aihara, *Acid and Alkaline* (The George Ohsawa Macrobiotic Foundation, 1971).

Toni Roberts Beard et al, *Healthwise Handbook* (Healthwise, Inc, 1976).

"Benign Alternative," *Off Our Backs*, May 1974.

Boston Women's Health Book Collective, *The New Our Bodies, Ourselves -- A Book by and for Women* (Simon and Schuster, 1984).

Gail Sforza Brewer, *The Pregnancy-After-30 Workbook* (Rodale Press, 1978).

Adelle Davis, *Let's Get Well* (Harcourt, Brace and World, 1965).

Rachel Farell, "Ask the Midwives," *The Practicing Midwife*, 1, No. 4.

Martindale, *The Extra Pharmacopoeia*, 26th edition, edited by Normal W. Blacow (The Pharmaceutical Press, 1972).

Harold Rosenberg, M.D., and A. N. Feldsamen, Ph.D., *The Doctor's Book of Vitamin Therapy, Megavitamins for Health* (G. P. Putnam's Sons, 1974).

Gerald N. Robenburg, *Compendium of Pharmaceuticals and Specialties*, 13th edition (Canadian Pharmaceutical Association, 1978).

Donald M. Vickery, M.D. and James F. Fries, M.D., *Take Care of Yourself, A Consumer's Guide to Medical Care* (Addison-Wesley Publishing Co., 1976).

Phyllis S. Williams, R.N., *Nourishing Your Unborn Child* (Avon Books, 1982).

Chapter Four
Preparing for Childbirth

I've experienced three births (including one stillbirth), each in a different setting.

The first was in 1966, at a large metropolitan hospital, with the most modern equipment and professional care. It was a miserable experience. My husband was "allowed" to be with me, but I couldn't bring anyone else, and I didn't know the doctors or the nurses. The doctors were cold and insensitive, and their exams were frequent and painful.

They put an I.V. in my arm, which prevented me from walking around and made it difficult to do effleurage on my abdomen (effleurage is a comforting circular massage, which eases the contractions). I'd already been in labor at home for twenty-four hours and my waters had broken, and they said there was a danger of infection, so they'd have to give me pitocin to speed up the labor. The pitocin intensified the contractions, which made them quite painful. The doctor said my pelvis was too small for the size of my baby's head and they'd probably have to do a cesarean. He insisted on taking x-rays, which I knew were dangerous for my baby.

After eight hours in the hospital, I was literally trembling with fear. The contractions had become quite painful, and it felt good to scream, but the nurse would "shush" me. Every few minutes she'd come in and say, "Wouldn't you like something for the pain, dear?" until the pain became so unbearable that I finally let them give me Demerol. Ten minutes later they took another x-ray and announced that I seemed to be progressing after all, and they would "let" me push my baby out. But it would be a forceps delivery, and they wouldn't allow my husband in the delivery room.

When my son was born, he was beautiful and alert and we looked each other in the eyes and I felt happy, even though they took him away "to clean him" before I could hold him.

My second baby was delivered at home, by a midwife. It was a beautiful experience. I was surrounded by loving, caring people. My young son was there with us. I was encouraged to follow my intuition, and I could make whatever noises I wanted to make, and I drank the teas I wanted to drink. I had control over my environment and the pace of my labor. When I felt like being alone, this was easily accommodated. I felt in tune with my body.

This beautiful birthing experience was my one consolation when my baby was born dead. It was not the midwife's fault: The baby had been dead inside for three days (according to the coroner's report). I didn't feel that having the baby at home endangered me or the baby in any way. I have my own understanding about why my baby died, and I accept her death. It was incredibly painful, but I accept it. People go to great lengths to avoid death, often creating badly damaged children instead. If we were not so terribly afraid of death, we could allow women and couples to make their own choices about where they want to have their babies, and with whom.

Yet I know that most people do not feel that way. My husband, for example (who is a nurse), persuaded me to have a clinic delivery with our third child. We found a wonderful doctor who had a clinic in a beautiful setting outside of town. He worked with a midwife who was my friend.

We arrived at the clinic half an hour before our baby was born (not intentionally). I had this baby on my own terms, with my husband, my friend, and my son, and it was almost as good as being at home. When my baby was born, he was put on my belly, and soon he was nursing at my breast, which helped bring on the contractions to deliver the placenta. Then we all had a feast (my husband brought lots of food), and we went home two hours later.

These experiences have reinforced my basic feelings that having a baby at home, under excellent conditions is the ultimate experience. Still, having a baby at a clinic under optimum conditions can be delightful. And despite my negative experience, having a baby in a hospital can be wonderful. The most important thing is having the baby.

WHO WILL BE AT THE BIRTH?

The Midwife or Labor Coach. A good midwife or labor coach will follow you through your prenatal visits, be there with you all through your labor and delivery, and then do postnatal visits to make sure that you and your baby are in good health.

Try to find a well-informed midwife or labor coach who works in collaboration with physicians and who can help you make decisions that feel good to you. This person should have skills to advise you during pregnancy and birth on how to avoid unnecessary interventions. She or he should be able to detect variations from normal and to inform you of your choices. If you do go to a hospital, this person should be able to go with you and stay with you until the baby is born.

In North America, we associate midwife-attended births with home births, but more and more nurse-midwives are practicing in hospitals. Other countries are more progressive *and safer* in providing various options for women.

In The Netherlands, for example, where they have the second lowest mortality rate in the world (the United States is fifteenth on the list), three times as many babies are born at home as in the hospital. Part of their success with home births they attribute to their selection process. Many women are screened out before their deliveries. And then, a significant part of midwifery training is to discern whether a mother or a baby are entering into a compromised situation when transfer to a hospital would be timely.

There is a model for this kind of birthing in North America. During a fifty-three-year period when the maternal mortality rate averaged 34 per 10,000 births, statistics from the Frontier Nursing Service in Kentucky (well-known for its training of highly competent nurse-midwives) showed that over the same period they lost only six mothers in 10,000 births (half of these were home deliveries). During the next twenty-six years of home and hospital experience, the Frontier Nursing Service delivered 10,000 babies with *no* maternal deaths.

I strongly advise that you have a midwife or labor coach with you throughout your labor and delivery. If you can find a competent midwife (whether she or he is a nurse-midwife or a lay midwife), you may also want to have this person deliver your baby.

The Doctor. It is a great pleasure to find a doctor who is warm, supportive, relaxed, and who enjoys being at deliveries. I've experienced working with such doctors, and they were well-loved by the birthing women and the midwives who worked with them.

Unfortunately, these doctors were usually not well-loved by their fellow-doctors. There is a lot of resistance in the medical profession against midwifery and home births. Birthing is a competitive business, and it is not in their best financial interest to encourage the competition. Consequently, many of these wonderful doctors have been severely harassed, and some of them have lost hospital privileges. So it has become increasingly difficult for midwives to find doctors who will provide back-up medical services for them.

When selecting a doctor, try to find someone you feel comfortable with. It's important that you feel comfortable about asking questions and describing how *you* want your delivery to be without feeling foolish. Inquire about the doctor's attitude about episiotomies, inducing or speeding up labor, squatting and different positions during delivery, and whatever issues are important to you. Even if you are planning a home delivery with a midwife, it's important to have a doctor for back-up. If you have a midwife or labor coach, ask this person to recommend a good doctor.

The Father. For some couples, it's essential for the father to be present at the birth. There is no substitute for the joyful bonding that occurs with a newborn baby. And it's extremely strengthening to a woman to have her partner truly *with* her as she experiences the tremendous activity in her body during labor and childbirth. A man who provides a hand to hold, eye contact, a sympathetic ear, and massage when it's needed is more valuable than he can imagine.

But not every man is cut out for the rigors of childbirth. Some men get queasy at the sight of blood. Some men can't stand to see their women in pain. So it's best for the man to decide if he really wants to be there.

If you decide that you want your partner and anyone else to be present throughout your labor and delivery, be sure to make such arrangements with the hospital of your choice beforehand, even if you just want to use the hospital as back-up for a home delivery.

Your Friend(s). For many women, it is indispensable to have a loving female friend to give her support through her labor — especially a woman who has given birth herself. At home, you can decide who will be present at your labor. If you want your two best friends as well as your partner and your kids, that's usually okay. You and your birth attendant(s) can work that out together.

Whoever comes to a birth should be more than spectators; they should be able to provide practical support as well as mental and physical support. Labor is an incredible exposure, and the mother should invite only people she can completely relax with.

There's a lot of physical work involved in delivering a baby and cleaning up afterwards, plus there are all the other domestic chores surrounding the birth. For this reason, it's a good idea at a home birth to have an assistant (who may be a close friend or relative of the mother's) to help with the chores and to give support as needed. As one midwife put it, "It's good to have people who are humble enough to wash dishes, even if they didn't get any dirty."

Be discriminating about who to invite to your birth. If you're not good at saying no, the whole neighborhood may drop by while you're in labor. Most midwives find that when there are a lot of people at a birth, the woman in labor tends to become self-conscious and may experience a kind of stage fright that leads to uterine inertia. Such births too often end up at the hospital, at which point labor proceeds smoothly.

Children. Sometimes children want to be at the delivery, or their parent(s) want them to be. A birth can be very exciting and sometimes overwhelming.

Dr. Marshall Klaus, the author of *Bonding*, recommends discouraging children under four years of age from attending births. He says they are less likely to ask questions about what they do not understand, and they are still dependent on their mothers for emotional support. He does not encourage having children present. Midwife Ina May Gaskin points out that a mother needs all her energy and attention focused on her own body, and a child can be a serious distraction for her.

Dr. Michael Odent emphasizes the importance of the woman who is in labor being as nearly uninhibited as possible, to enable her to become more instinctive and to follow the lead of her body. Having a small child present will pull her out of her concentration on herself and may be a drain on her energies.

Some parts of labor and childbirth are distressing to some children. But if they are well-prepared, these effects can be minimized. Though children respond differently during the various stages of the experience, sounds made by the mother are often disturbing to the children unless they've been prepared to expect unusual sounds and can interpret them as a positive sign.

Some mothers have found it very satisfying to have their teenage daughters present at their births. If there is a close tie between the mother and daughter, this can be a beautiful experience.

If a child is there, arrange for an adult—someone the child already knows and trusts—to be present just to be with the child and answer questions and give attention when needed (or, if necessary, to take the child away). Make it clear that the child can leave at any time. Be sure there is a separate room for the child with toys and food.

It is far more important for children to see their new brother or sister soon after the birth than to actually be present for the event. But many hospitals do not allow children as visitors. This is a tragic loss to the bonding that is so essential within a family. And when a child is kept away from his or her mother, there is likely to be resentment toward the new baby. If the child visits the mother and baby in the hospital, Klaus recommends that someone else should hold the baby at first, to allow the mother to give undivided attention to the child she has not seen. Then the new baby can be introduced to its sibling.

ARE YOU "HIGH-RISK"?

When a woman is categorized as high-risk, this automatically implies that she should not deliver at home, and that she is a possible candidate for various "life-saving" interventions. Consequently, "high-risk" for many women translates to "at a high risk of having a cesarean section."

There is a lot of disagreement over what constitutes high risk, and many midwives and some medical people are reluctant to attach that label to healthy women who fall into the "high-risk" pigeonholes. There are arguments about which categories of so-called high risk women might respond better to the supportive, calm environment of a loving home—or clinic.

Many high-risk conditions are indications that the newborn might be at risk. Then the chances of saving the baby may be improved if you can be in a hospital where the baby can be put into intensive care if necessary. If you anticipate such circumstances, then try to find a supportive hospital that honors the importance of bonding.

The following conditions are usually considered high risk. The ones marked with an asterisk (*) are debatable.

Overweight*
Malnourished

Anemic
Diabetic
Emotionally unstable*
Severely stressed*
Rh negative woman mated to Rh positive man
Being over forty years old or under eighteen*
Having first babies at age thirty-five or over*
Drug addicted
Heavy smokers
Heavy drinkers

Premature labor (less than thirty-seven weeks)
Overdue labor (about two to three weeks)*
Waters breaking more than twelve hours before labor starts or
    twenty-four hours before the baby is born (because of the pos-
    sibility of infection)*
Serious illnesses, such as tuberculosis or pneumonia
Heart or circulatory disorders, including high blood pressure
Kidney disorders or urinary tract infections
Active herpes lesions or gonorrhea
Toxoplasmosis
Having had more than six children or abortions*
Previous cesarean deliveries*
Android (manlike) pelvis*
Incompetent cervix
Relatives with severe genetic defects

Babies who seem to be small for their dates
Breech presentations (though a frank breech is less high-risk)*
Twins*

HOME BIRTH

The safety of a home birth depends on how well prepared you are, who is present at the birth and how much experience they've had, and what kind of equipment is available. A well-trained and well-equipped midwife or doctor can provide the same I.V.s, oxygen, and much of the emergency equipment that a hospital or clinic provides. At home, there will be less exposure to staph, strep, and other disease organisms that are common to hospitals. But you will need to provide a clean room for the delivery. If your house is too chaotic, you may be endangering yourself and your baby.

If you have a well-trained midwife and the back-up of a doctor with hospital privileges, a home birth may be safer than a hospital delivery.

Many women and men are more contented and relaxed at home. They feel secure and confident in their own environment. This is important when giving birth, because relaxation is essential. Certainly the intimacy of close physical contact which many couples enjoy during labor is difficult if not impossible in most hospitals. Giving birth can be a very sensual experience, but that rarely happens in the sterile surroundings of a hospital, and in the company of an unfamiliar medical staff.

If your home is far from a hospital, especially if it is along bumpy roads, or roads that can be dangerous in winter (if the baby is due in winter), you'd be wise to plan to give birth at a friend's house in town or at a birth center, if one is available.

Medical establishments often claim that hospital births are far safer than home births. This is based on misleading statistics that include premature births which were not intended to occur at home, late miscarriages, and births that took place with no trained attendant. When the statistics are limited to births that were planned to occur at home, with a trained attendant, birthing at home is actually safer for the mother and baby who are not high risk. In fact, some studies suggest that even the mother who is at risk is better off birthing at home or in a clinic.

British statistician Marjorie Tew reports in the *Journal of the Royal College of General Practitioners 1985* that perinatal mortality (infant death just before and after birth) was lower at home or clinic for *all* risk groups. It could be argued that there would be less deaths at home, since women would be transferred to the hospital if the babies were believed to be in danger. But this is only a further argument for home or clinic delivery by trained attendants, because part of the training is knowing when to consult a doctor and when to go to the hospital. Unfortunately, too many hospitals have closed their doors to midwives, and also to doctors who do home deliveries. I believe that it is *only* this lack of cooperation that makes home deliveries more dangerous.

Dr. Lewis Mehl, director of The Institute for Childbirth and Family Research in Berkeley, did a study comparing 421 home births attended by noncertified midwives (judged by the investigators to be experienced and knowledgeable) with an equal number of hospital births attended by physicians. This study yielded better outcomes for the midwives. However, when only the less interventionist half of the physicians were compared with the midwives, few significant differences were found.

Sometimes there is a death at a home birth, or a significant mistake is made by a midwife. Our culture seems to feel more comfortable with deaths that occur in hopitals. People can say to themselves, "We did everything we could." It used to be this way with people who had terminal illnesses. The hospice movement has introduced the concept that people should be allowed to die at home when that is their choice. Similarly, our children will not be allowed to be born at home until we can accept — and legalize — the possibility that a rare child may die during a home birth, just as they do in hospitals.

Preparing for a Home Delivery*

About a week before the due date, freshen up your birth room. Sweep and mop the floor and dust the furniture and surfaces. You may want to use vinegar in water (two tablespoons per quart) or Lysol or some other disinfectant. Straighten out the room by getting rid of irrelevant things. Keep all surfaces clear.

A simple procedure to provide the amount of cleanliness required for most births is to double-wrap birth materials in two paper bags, rolling down the tops of both bags together and stapling or taping them closed. Then put the bags in the oven at 200 degrees F. for two hours. To prevent scorching, place a pan of water in the bottom of the oven, or wrap the bag in tinfoil, with the dull side out.

Materials should remain relatively sterile for two weeks. If they haven't been used by that time, simply place the unopened bags in the oven for another two hours. If you haven't time for this procedure, use freshly laundered materials that have been dried in a hot dryer, or sun-dried, or ironed. Be sure that all materials used for vaginal exams and for dealing with torn or cut edges have been prepared by one of these methods.

These precautions are for your own safety, because when your cervix dilates during childbirth, your uterus (which is normally closed) opens onto the place where the placenta was attached. This exposes your blood vessels and makes you vulnerable to infection. If the surroundings are very clean, there's nothing to worry about. You are actually less liable to get an infection in a clean home than in a hospital because there are so many disease organisms in hospitals.

The following materials should be on hand at a home delivery. Bulleted items are also useful for a clinic or hospital delivery. Of course, the midwife will bring additional supplies.

- **Firm bed**. There are various positions for birthing your baby, but it's difficult to know which position is most comfortable for you until you're in the final stage of labor. You may want to deliver by squatting on the floor, with disposable pads underneath you. But there's always a chance that you'll want to deliver in bed. If your bed sags, put a board or piece of plywood under the mattress, because during delivery the fluid might gather in a pool, which could be dangerous for the baby, since most babies are born face down. If you can't get a firm bed or find a board, you can deliver at the edge of the bed with your feet and back supported.
- **Plastic cover for the bed**.
- **Two sets of sheets**. Put one set under the plastic, so a clean bed will be ready after the birth.

*Written in consultation with Marion Toepke, nurse-midwife and nurse-practitioner.

- **Disposable pads**. These will go under you at the time of delivery to catch the fluids. You can make these yourself by using twelve thicknesses of newspaper, with an old sheet or cloth sewn on top. It's a good idea to have two full-size pads made from fully opened newspapers and six half-size pads made from newspapers that have been folded once. Or use disposable incontinent pads, or disposable diapers — preferably without elastic legs — toddler size. These disposables are also useful to wear if your membranes have ruptured early in labor, and for the first twenty-four hours after giving birth.
- **Maxi pads**. To wear after the first twenty-four hours.
- **Sterile towels**. Two small towels, in case stitches are required. (Usually the midwife will provide her own materials to create a sterile field.)
- **Freshly laundered towels**. About six towels that have been laundered within the last two weeks and then dried in a hot drier and wrapped in a clean plastic or paper bag. (After two weeks, launder again.)
- **Receiving blankets**. About six, freshly laundered.
- **Good light source**. You need a light that can be focused and directed; a gooseneck lamp works well. Be sure to have an extra bulb.
- **Small table**. To set supplies on, at about the height of the bed.
- **Commode**. If your birth room is not right next to the bathroom, it's a good idea to provide some kind of commode so you can pass urine as well as stool while in labor without having to walk far. A large pot with a lid and toilet paper will do. The birth room at one birth center has a Chinese screen behind which sits an old-fashioned chamber pot.
- **Enema**. This is good to have in case it's needed. An enema bag with warm tap water will suffice. Or you may prefer a disposable Fleet's phosphate enema, which can be purchased at any drugstore.
- **Heating pad or hot water bottle***. To help relieve aches and pains. If this is not available, have some extra towels on hand. These can be heated in the oven or dipped in hot water and then wrung out and applied to your back or abdomen (cover with flannel to keep the heat in).
- **Lip salve***. Your lips may get dried out if you're doing a lot of heavy breathing.
- **Oil for massage***. Especially if you have back labor, you will welcome a good massage.
- **Unopened bottle of vegetable oil**. To apply to your perineum to help it to stretch, just before your baby is born.
- **Herb teas***. As described in chapter 5 under "Nourishment During Labor." If you won't be at home, these can be prepared beforehand and taken in a thermos or jar.
- **Two pots with tight lids**. To sterilize water for washing your vagina before and after giving birth. A big and little pot will enable the midwife to keep a small pot by the bedside and a large pot on the stove, so

she'll be more likely to get the right temperature when she needs it. Alternately, you could provide a large thermos.

- **Food or drink to keep your blood sugar up***. Appropriate foods and liquids are discussed in chapter 5 under "Nourishment During Labor."
- **Oral thermometer**. For the mother.
- **Rectal thermometer**. For the baby.
- **Alcohol and cotton balls**. For cord care.
- **Antiseptic solution**. You can use a standard antiseptic, or you can make your own by adding one cup of boiling water to one teaspoon goldenseal and a half teaspoon of myrrh. Cover and steep for five minutes, then strain through cheesecloth. Keep refrigerated.
- **Warm place for your baby***. Now that research has confirmed the importance of skin-to-skin contact, many progressive hospitals and birth centers are providing a heat panel so that the newborn naked baby can enjoy skin-to-skin contact with its mother. But your own body gives off plenty of warmth, and you and your baby can both be covered by a soft quilt or a warm receiving blanket. To warm the receiving blanket, put it in a closed paper bag and place it in an oven at 200 degrees for about ten minutes.
- **Diapers, diaper pins, and baby clothes***.
- **Slippers and robe***. For the mother.
- **Food for after the birth (or during)***. Even if your partner and/or friends are eager to cook for you, it's nice to have at least one hearty meal in your freezer, because after the birth, everyone's so excited they usually don't feel like doing anything that distracts them from this miraculous new being. Don't be afraid of eating a hearty meal after all the work you've done. Just follow your intuition about what and how much to eat.

BIRTH CENTERS

A good birth center can provide a warm, clean, comfortable environment that may be more relaxing than a hospital. For some women, it is more relaxing than their home, since it relieves them of responsibilities.

The personnel at a birth center are likely to let you have your birth on your own terms: You can have whom you want at your birth, you can eat lightly if you wish while in labor, you can prepare herb teas, you can birth in whatever position you're most comfortable, you can be alone with your partner, there can be physical closeness between you and your partner or nudity (many women find clothes constricting during labor).

There *may* be more equipment available at a birth center, but most of the equipment at a center can be provided by a well-equipped midwife. Some doctors feel more secure working in this environment, so you're more likely to have a doctor at your birth (and doctors who work in birth centers are usually non-interventionist). If your home is more than twenty minutes from a hospital, a birth center could put you in a more strategic location. If you have any reason to expect a difficult birth, this is certainly a good compromise between the hospital and the home, but unfortunately, you may not be allowed to have your baby in a birth center if you are considered high risk.

The Siuslaw Rural Health Center near Eugene, Oregon (a clinic which I helped to start), is located next to a beautiful river with a patio and mimosa trees. The birth room is a big room with sliding glass doors that look out over the river. It provides an important service, because many of the women who live in this rural area want to birth at home, but they live over an hour from the nearest hospital. The clinic is only ten minutes from the hospital.

We wanted this room to feel warm and homey, so we commissioned a local carpenter to make a hand-carved wooden headboard and a lovely wooden rocking chair. There are gifts that have been donated by grateful people who have used and cherish this birth room: a handmade quilt, a woven "God's eye," and paintings on the wall.

We were fortunate to have a nurse-midwife and some lay midwives that she trained and a supportive doctor. The midwife delivered the babies and the doctor assisted only when needed. On rare occasions, the women were transferred to the local hospital.

Some birth centers are located as a wing of the hospital. For example, Mount Zion Hospital in San Francisco has a birth center. In this environment birth can be conducted with the assumption that it will be natural, without intervention. Since doctors who work in such centers tend to prefer natural births, this helps to create the kind of environment that will further that outcome.

Statistics from Mount Zion show that emergency situations arose in 1.5 percent of births where it was believed that the mother or the baby might have been in danger of dying if the birth had occurred at home. These included a case of thick meconium which was discovered too late to move the mother, but which endangered the baby and required endotracheal intubation for resuscitation of the infant. Another was an infant with congenital heart disease. And others included mothers with significant postpartum hemorrhage.

HOSPITAL BIRTH

Hospital practices have changed radically over the last ten years. In some cases, they have changed for the better — partly because women have demanded reforms, but also because a new generation of nurses and doctors have, at times, offered a more humanitarian form of health care. In other cases, they have changed for the worse — mostly because a new technology has revolutionized birth practices, and because the high price of the equipment and the fear of malpractice suits have contributed to the overuse of this technology (to justify the additional expense).

There are different kinds of hospitals. Some are friendly and others are unfriendly; some encourage the patient's involvement in her own care and others assume complete authority; some are non-interventionist and others intervene a great deal; some are well-staffed and others are understaffed. Whether you *plan* to have your child at home, in a birth center, or in a hospital, visit your local hospital(s) *before* your delivery. The hospital is a necessary back-up to any birthing procedure, and in case of an emergency, it's better to know what to expect.

Most hospitals will give you a tour of their facilities. Ask questions: Do they give routine episiotomies? What is their cesarean rate? Will they allow your partner in the delivery room? Will they allow your labor coach and your friend? What procedures do they follow for the baby after birth? Will they let you keep your baby with you to nurse on demand? If the baby is kept in a nursery at night, will they bring the baby to you to nurse when he or she wakes up? Will your children be able to visit their new brother or sister?

There are vast differences among hospitals. For example, in the state of New York, cesarean rates vary from less than one percent in one hospital to more than 25 percent in another. So if you think you may want or need a hospital delivery, and if you can choose between hospitals, then study the statistics, policies, and reputations of each.

Some small-town hospitals have very little emergency equipment and the staff may be underqualified and overworked. Or they may be highly qualified and more experienced in the art of delivery, and the lack of expensive equipment may be a blessing, since doctors who have it tend to use it. However, if you have reason to believe that you or your baby may require some of the more modern technology, you may want to travel to a larger hospital, or have your baby at a home or birth center that is close to one.

If you're being seen by a doctor you like, you'll want to know in which hospital(s) he or she has admitting privileges. If you have a midwife, you'll want to know if the hospital of your choice will allow your midwife to stay with you throughout your labor and delivery. In fact, some hospitals allow nurse-midwives to deliver normal births.

But regardless of who actually delivers your baby, it is invaluable to have a midwife with you throughout your labor and delivery — especially if you are considered high-risk, because you want to avoid any unnecessary interventions. It is essential to have someone you trust; someone who is well-informed. This person can help you to evaluate whether suggested interventions are actually necessary or if they are just for the convenience of the medical staff.

For some mothers, it's a great relief to leave the children and responsibilities of home for a few days. If these mothers remain at home, they are likely to be on their feet too soon — cooking, cleaning, and taking care of their families. If you don't have someone who can take care of you and your house and family for at least three days (and preferably for two weeks after your baby is born), then a hospital (or birth center) may be the only way to give yourself the time and space you need for optimum recovery.

If you plan to have a home birth, but you end up in the hospital, this can be very disappointing; but remember that a complicated childbirth can be a matter of life and death. Ultimately, the most important thing is the health and safety of you and your child. And if all goes well, you can leave the hospital soon after the delivery.

Routine Hospital Procedures

These procedures will vary from one hospital to another. In researching hospitals, inquire about their policies on the issues that concern you. If the staff is unwilling to discuss their policies, don't be intimidated. This will give you valuable information, because one of the most important requirements for good health care is a willingness to keep you informed and to include you in the decision-making.

The following procedures are common in many hospitals.

Masking

If your partner or anybody else wants to be present at your delivery, they may be required to wear a mask and gown. As long as everyone is healthy, there's no reason for it. At one birth center, the head nurse screens everyone who is present at the delivery, and later, whoever visits the newborn, to be sure that no one is ill.

Shaving or Prepping

The pubic hair is sometimes shaved, presumably to prevent infection, since hair cannot be sterilized. However, no scientific study has shown that shaving reduces the rate of infection. In fact, there is a greater risk of lacerations or abrasions which can lead to infections. This practice probably dates back to when lice were rampant.

Enemas

These are used routinely in some hospitals, yet many women don't need them. The body's natural reaction to labor is for the bowels to empty themselves. But if you've been constipated, you may have some trouble. A full bowel can cause painful contractions. The uterus is between the bowel and the bladder, so a full bowel or bladder can interfere with labor. There's also the possibility of pushing through fecal matter while you're pushing out your baby, which seems to be more distressing to obstetricians than to midwives (this does happen occasionally, though no harm is done). Enemas are distasteful to many women, and I believe that the choice of whether or not to have one should be up to you.

Fasting

North American women are unique in being deprived of food and sometimes fluids while they labor. The rationale is that in case general anesthesia is needed, you might vomit and then inhale the contents of your stomach, which could be fatal. However, women in other countries eat lightly and drink during labor and many of these countries have lower fatality rates than the U.S. They also have fewer cesareans.

I.V.s (Intravenous Feedings)

Many hospitals routinely give I.V.s to women who have been in labor for a long time to prevent the blood sugar from going too low, to prevent dehydration, and to make it easier to administer emergency drugs. I.V. is short for intravenous, and it refers to the small tube that is inserted into the vein of the arm at one end and attached to a bottle at the other end. The bottle holds glucose (sugar) and water, but it can also hold medications.

The sugar water used in I.V.s is devoid of protein. Sugar and honey are considered high energy sources, but energy is measured in calories, and fat has almost twice as many calories as sugars and starches, so fat supplies twice as much energy. A good substitute for an I.V. is yogurt made from whole milk with honey or molasses. By combining a natural sugar with fat, you get a quick energy boost, and by the time the effect starts to wear off, the fat from the yogurt — which takes much longer to digest — starts giving you energy, which lasts for a longer time.

The I.V. also keeps a line open for the easy administration of drugs in case of an emergency. But most emergencies do not occur without warning, and generally there is plenty of time to set up an I.V. if it is needed. Puncturing your blood vessel (and there may be several punctures) increases the chance of contracting hospital-borne infections.

The I.V. contributes to keeping you on your back, attached by a tube to a heavy bottle, making it difficult to enjoy massaging your belly, or walking around easily, exercising, or feeling comfortable squatting or changing positions. All of these limitations contribute to difficulties during childbirth, as explained below.

There are times when an I.V. is vital and if you have a labor coach, this person can help you to determine if the I.V. should be used. But the routine use of I.V.s should be discouraged.

Supine Position (On Your Back)

Throughout history women have given birth leaning, squatting, holding onto ropes or onto their men, bracing their feet against the wall or against a piece of furniture. But never, until men took over the delivery of babies in the 1800s, did women give birth on their backs. No other animal has assumed such an improbable and powerless position for birthing.

The only advantage of the supine position (or lithotomy — with feet in stirrups) is that it's convenient for the obstetrician. The weight of your uterus presses down on major blood vessels, interfering with circulation and decreasing blood pressure. This diminishes the oxygen supply to your baby, which increases the risk of fetal distress and asphyxia. In such an uncomfortable position and with so little control over movement, the pain increases, leading to the use of painkillers. Since the baby must work against gravity, labor is slow, adequate dilation of the cervix may not take place, and you may be diagnosed as having a pelvis that is too small for a normal vaginal delivery. This leads to forceps or cesarean deliveries.

Induction and Speeding Up Labor
Doctors may decide to induce labor for reasons ranging from a serious concern for the mother or baby to a convenience on the part of the doctor. Hospital space is limited and expensive, so hospitals rarely allow women to labor at their own pace. On the other hand, there are legitimate indications for inductions, including Rh isoimmunization, diabetes, preeclampsia, high blood pressure, kidney disease, and growth retardation.

There are two methods of induction and speeding up labor: amniotomy ("breaking the bag of waters") and oxytocin (or pitocin).

Amniotomy. With this procedure, the bag of waters is ruptured. This is painful, especially if the cervix is not "ripe," which occurs when the lower portion of the cervix expands and becomes very thin, making it less sensitive to pain.

Throughout pregnancy, the baby floats in amniotic fluid. The amniotic sac holds both the baby and the fluid, keeping them sterile and cushioned. When the sac is broken, the contents are exposed to external bacteria, making infection more likely. When the bag of waters breaks naturally, the lining keeps producing fluid, and the baby's head acts as a seal to prevent the fluid from escaping through the cervix, so there is still enough cushioning to protect the baby's head from bumping up against the hard cervix during labor.

When the bag of waters is ruptured artificially, labor is speeded up by only about twenty to thirty minutes. When the membranes are ruptured artificially, there's a greater chance of traumatic injury to the baby because it diminishes the cushion of fluid which protects its head during childbirth. There's a higher incidence of umbilical cord compression without the extra padding. This may lead to fetal distress because the baby's oxygen supply is compromised — which is an indication for cesarean.

Another reason for breaking the bag of waters is to observe the amniotic fluid. If the baby has been traumatized, the anal sphincter will relax (as in, "you scared the shit out of him"), and meconium will be released into the amniotic fluid. Meconium is the first elimination of the baby; it's dark green, mucilaginous, and sticky. Ordinarily, amniotic fluid is clear, odorless, and watery. The meconium turns the fluid a greenish or brown color, and it may give it an odor or make it thicker.

There is some danger that the baby may aspirate or inhale the meconium, making it difficult to breathe. Therefore, meconium in the amniotic fluid is often considered an indication that a cesarean should be performed. However, if the baby has normal heart tones, there's no cause for alarm. One study showed no significant difference in outcome for babies with or without meconium — even when the meconium was thick and solid.

Doctors will caution you about the danger of infection if your bag of waters breaks prematurely, but the greatest danger comes from repeated vaginal exams which introduce bacteria into the vagina. Women with longer labors, especially those who labor in hospitals, are more likely to have frequent vaginal exams — particularly when an internal fetal monitor is being used, since more exams are needed in order to check the equipment.

Oxytocin. Pitocin or oxytocin is used to induce labor or to strengthen uterine contractions during labor. It is administered through the I.V. Oxytocin is normally produced by the pituitary gland, but it can also be synthetically prepared.

Oxytocin-induced contractions are more frequent, painful, and grabbing than the wave-like contractions of non-drug induced labor. Consequently, this form of induction usually leads to the use of painkillers. According to British figures, 50 percent of noninduced mothers deliver without painkillers, but only 8 percent of induced mothers can avoid them.

Ordinarily, oxygen does not reach the baby during contractions. This doesn't seem to be a problem with normal contractions, but harsh, prolonged, induced contractions can lead to fetal distress — an indication for a cesarean.

Induction is sometimes recommended because the pregnancy has exceeded forty weeks, but it often happens that the due date was miscalculated, and the result is a premature baby, who may have respiratory distress syndrome or other problems which can lead to prolonged hospitalization and interference with bonding.

Ultrasound
These waves of vibratory motion cannot be heard by the human ear. They travel through water and bounce off surfaces in their path, like an echo. The echo creates a picture, much as a bat uses radar to "see." Until recently, patients were assured that this process was entirely harmless. Now researchers are questioning its safety and some are urging that it be used only with extreme discretion. Three forms of ultrasound are used during pregnancy: the Doptone, the external fetal monitor, and diagnostic ultrasound.

Doptone. The Doptone is a harmless-looking little box, which has virtually replaced the old-fashioned fetoscope and stethoscope. It is a fairly irresistible piece of equipment which seems to allow parents to hear their baby's heartbeat. Actually, the Doptone emits a continuous wave of ultrasound which is directed toward the fetus's moving blood in the placenta. Some women have reported that their babies jump when the Doptone is used. One study showed that fetuses displayed increased activity after five minutes of exposure to the Doptone.

The Doptone is probably the least potentially harmful of the ultrasound devices because it has a very low intensity and is generally used for a short time. To minimize any possible risks, *The Practicing Midwife* recommends the following guidelines for midwives (this magazine is published by The Farm in Tennessee, well-known for its non-interventionist home births).

1) Avoid use during the first trimester except when medically indicated (in case of suspected missed abortion, etc.)

2) Avoid use for extended periods. Use a conventional fetoscope when you can, but keep a Doppler on hand for when you might need one, particularly in the second stage of labor when you need to determine the fetal heart rate and make fast decisions.

3) Use an instrument with the lowest possible power output. If you're buying a Doppler stethoscope, ask for specifications as to the instrument's output. Most instruments on the market have a very low output (under 25 mW/cm2).

In most cases, the Doptone really isn't needed. By the twentieth week, a baby's heartbeat can be heard with a stethoscope or fetoscope.

Diagnostic Ultrasound. This new diagnostic tool has replaced x-rays by allowing physicians to study the inner contents of the body through beaming in high-frequency sound waves. When they echo back from different surfaces and densities, they're reflected as a series of dots which form into moving pictures. During pregnancy, an image of the embryo or fetus can be observed.

Private physicians are now purchasing sonographic devices for their offices, and many of them are eager to use their new equipment. Doctors often tell women, "Let's just get an ultrasound so I'll know what position your baby is in." Please be cautious. Let's not make our babies and ourselves into guinea pigs. As Doreen Liebeskind, M.D., points out, when a female child receives ultrasound in utero, all of her cells are exposed, as are all of her eggs for the next generation. Premature ovulation has been reported by Testart after female babies receive ovarian ultrasonography in utero.

M. E. Stratmeyer, research scientist at the Bureau of Radiological Health of the Food and Drug Administration writes, "We need more information on both safety and efficacy before we can endorse the unrestrained use of ultrasound during pregnancy. . . . one hopes it will be used prudently while we await definite answers as to biological effects."

The results of diagnostic ultrasound are frequently inaccurate. Even twins — and once triplets — have gone undiagnosed by ultrasound. One of the most common overuses of ultrasound is for estimating gestational age. This is very difficult to determine, particularly during the third trimester, because of variations in growth rate. So this form of diagnosis frequently leads to unnecessary cesareans in which the baby is sometimes premature, and therefore more at risk because of the cesarean.

Ultrasound is reliable for determining fetal position, but a doctor or midwife with sensitive hands can do that. It can be used to determine the position of the placenta before birth, but this can lead to unnecessary cesareans, since the placenta often moves out of the way on its own. It is routinely used before amniocentesis, but one might think very seriously about whether amniocentesis is absolutely necessary — especially when so little is known about the effects of ultrasound when used in the first trimester, during the development of the internal organs.

There is no conclusive evidence that diagnostic levels of ultrasound are definitely harmful to humans, but there are plenty of animal studies which should lead us to use extreme caution. A study by Dr. Doreen Liebeskind strongly suggests chromosome breakage and the partial unwinding of the helix in DNA. Another study shows that ultrasound has the ability to interfere with normal development of the fruit fly. Still other animal studies show decreased clotting time, liver cell damage in mice, dilation of blood vessels, corneal erosion in the eyes, brain enzyme alterations, alteration in electrical activity (EEG) in the brain, delayed reflexes, emotional reactivity, and disruption of the spleen's ability to produce antibodies resulting in reduced immunology.

New drugs are required to pass stringent tests before being introduced for human use. Yet the same regulations do not apply to new equipment. The medical profession seems to take the attitude of "innocent until proven guilty." When it comes to newborn babies, this is a foolhardy policy. Stratmeyer and other researchers point out that the safety of ultrasound is based primarily on "clinical impressions." Since we cannot see any fetal abnormalities, we assume that there are none and never will be. He says, "There is little scientific evaluation of how effective ultrasound procedures are." This is confirmed by the American College of Obstetricians and Gynecologists (ACOG): "No well-controlled study has yet proved that routine scanning of all prenatal patients will improve the outcome of pregnancy."

Stratmeyer adds,

At the present time, we cannot take what we know about exposed human populations and say that ultrasound is safe or unsafe. . . . Most of the testing was done at birth. Delayed effects were not tested for. . . . most of the exposures in the earlier studies occurred during the second and third trimester, after the period of major organogenesis. Therefore, one would not expect to see fetal abnormalities. Now, however, there is a tendency to use ultrasound more in the first trimester.

The American Medical Association and the Food and Drug Administration are now cautioning against the unnecessary use of ultrasound in obstetrics. They are recommending that inquiries regarding the safety of diagnostic levels should not be met with assurances of safety.

In their book, *Silent Knife*, Nancy Wainer Cohen and Lois J. Estner suggest, "If diagnostic ultrasound is recommended, ask for full details: Why is it recommended? Would the results be absolutely accurate at this point in your pregnancy? Would the scan provide essential information that cannot be gathered any other way and which would then determine resultant care? What difference does it make of you already know your 'due date'?"

Electronic Fetal Heart Monitor. This instrument also works on the Doppler principle. Doppler observed that sound waves change in pitch or frequency according to movement — for example, when a train moves toward you, the sound of the train whistle gets higher in pitch, and then lower as the train moves away. By use of the Doppler effect, the electronic fetal monitor provides a continuous recording of the fetal heart tones. The baby is exposed to a continuous wave of ultrasound throughout labor.

With the indirect or external fetal monitor, you have electrodes on your abdomen and a belt to hold them on. With the internal fetal monitor, your bag of waters is broken (if it isn't already) and a wire is threaded into your uterus, where the electrodes are attached to your baby's scalp. Then the fetal heartbeat can be displayed on an oscilloscope screen. Another needle may be inserted into the baby's head to collect blood for oxygen analysis.

A baby would have to be very ill before a mother would allow anyone to stick anything into her its scalp. But the fear generated by the hospital setting causes women to give up their power. They are told that without the electronic fetal monitor, their babies would be at greater risk. Yet studies have shown that more electronically monitored women end up in the operating room with cesarean deliveries than women who are monitored with a stethoscope. *And there is no improvement in perinatal outcome* for babies delivered by cesarean.

Meanwhile, the mother is forced to stay on her back, which lowers her blood pressure and decreases the oxygen supply to her baby, which produces abnormalities in the baby's heart rate. So the electronic fetal monitor actually contributes to the distress it is supposed to monitor, which leads to an increase in cesarean sections.

Internal monitoring provides a possible route for the entry of bacteria into the amniotic fluid. There will be excessive vaginal exams simply to check the equipment. Infection rates in women who are internally monitored are double that of manually monitored women. The baby can also get infected through the scalp.

The external method is notorious for errors in measurement, and babies are frequently rescued from supposed fetal distress by emergency cesareans, only to be found in perfect health.

As Yvonne Brackbill points out in her excellent book, *Birth Trap*, the electronic fetal monitor is a very expensive piece of equipment, and it requires a lot of use to pay for itself. This may explain why its use is becoming routine, instead of being reserved for emergencies.

Episiotomy

This is a cut in the perineum (the area between the vagina and the anus), which enlarges the vaginal opening. After the birth, it is sutured. There is a belief among physicians that this operation will prevent "pelvic floor incompetence." But long-term follow-up data show no correlation between episiotomies and pelvic floor incompetence.

Another justification is that it avoids tearing the perineum as the baby's head emerges. It is ironic that one study found nine times as many severe tears in hospital deliveries as in home births, even though there were nine times as many episiotomies among the hospital deliveries. There are other ways of handling a birth which can help to prevent tearing (see "Perineal Massage" in chapter 5). If tearing does occur, it is usually not difficult to mend—though a severe tear requires skillful mending.

Medications

Although most doctors are not patient, they do like to feel useful, and they are well-trained in the administration of drugs. Although drugs are supposed to protect and help you, they are dangerous in themselves—for you and your baby. While it may be comforting to know that you have drugs as a back-up, you should know that one drug leads to another. Oxytocin (pitocin) will speed up your labor, but it will also create painful contractions, usually necessitating a narcotic. But the painkiller will make your baby groggy, so you may be given a narcotic antagonist.

Painkillers decrease your blood pressure, which diminishes the oxygen supply to the fetus, which may trigger an abnormal fetal heart rate, which often results in a cesarean. A baby's brain and central nervous system are very delicate. Obstetrical drugs cross the placenta and enter fetal circulation within minutes of their administration to the mother.

Narcotic drugs will decrease your mental alertness and interfere with maternal-infant bonding. They are often responsible for postpartum depression, which is a common complaint from women who deliver in hospitals, and rarely seen among women who deliver at home. Statistics of home deliveries in the United States (with and without physicians) show that deliveries without drugs range between 95 and 100 percent. By contrast, hospital deliveries with drugs come very close to 100 percent.

Why do midwives and non-intervenionist doctors rarely require these drugs? A skilled midwife or doctor has the gift of touch, encouragement, and a basic confidence in a woman's ability to birth her baby. In fact, there is no reason why midwives cannot be brought into the hospital, as they have been in Sweden, where midwives deliver most babies in hospitals. Sweden has the safest record of deliveries in the world.

There is nothing inherently bad about hospitals. But ironically, our current "life-saving" drugs and technology have made North America a relatively dangerous place to have a baby. On a world scale, the United States ranks fifteenth in fetal and maternal morbidity and mortality.

Forceps and Vacuum Extractions
In the United States, forceps or vacuum extractions are used in 5 to 20 percent of deliveries. There has been a decline in forceps deliveries as cesareans have gained in popularity, probably because forceps deliveries require more skill and present more danger of injury to the baby (and hence a greater danger of lawsuits to the physician).

Delayed Bonding
When a woman delivers at home or in a birth center, the baby is usually put on her belly, and then at her breast. She and the father and whoever else is present have an opportunity to exchange eye-to-eye and flesh-to-flesh contact with this new and impressionable being. After having been in relative sense-deprivation for nine months, this is a very exciting time, and this newborn person is going to make some assumptions about how life will be based on these first impressions. We want to provide the optimum love, warmth, and affection to these precious, perfectly new babies.

Most mothers have an intuitive desire to stay with their babies after the birth, and mothers who are deprived of their babies suffer from depression, guilt, and anger.

Through hypnosis, I've taken many of my clients back to the moment of their own birth, and those who were deprived of their mothers just after birth wondered if they were loved and cared about.

Hospitals and even cesarean deliveries do not necessarily have to deprive us of this essential bonding experience. In fact, most hospitals now offer lying-in facilities in which the mother and infant can remain together, instead of taking the baby to the nursery. Some facilities allow the father round-the-clock access, but very few allow admittance to siblings, who should be encouraged to bond with their newborn brothers and sisters, and who may otherwise resent having their mothers taken away from them.

It should be an inalienable human right for babies to be with their mothers after birth—unless the separation is truly essential for the health of either one—in which case, the parents should be included in making that decision.

CESAREANS *

Back in 1968, doctors were very cautious about performing a cesarean. The overall rate in the United States was 5 percent of all births. By 1978, over 15 percent of all deliveries were done by cesarean, and by 1982, the cesarean section rate for the United States was 18 percent — one of the highest rates of cesareans in the world. The United States has the most sophisticated equipment and technology, and yet cesareans are performed at twice the British rate and about four times the western European average.

Meanwhile, other countries with *lower* cesarean rates have significantly *lower* mortality rates — for both mothers and babies. What accounts for the rise in cesareans in North America?

The birth rate in North America has been decreasing, yet the number of obstetricians has been rising. In 1963, an obstetrician could expect to deliver (and bill) 261 patients in a year. By 1975, that number had dropped to 145 patients per year, and the figures are still falling. Doctors' fees for surgical delivery are about twice as high as for vaginal delivery, and that doesn't include all the extras.

In the old days, obstetricians were more skillful, yet they had less status in the eyes of their medical peers, and they commanded a relatively low level of income. The new obstetricians rank second only to the surgeons and anesthesiologists, and they command a similarly high level of income.

In the old days, an obstetrician was judged by how few cesareans were performed. Obstetrics was considered an art. An old-fashioned doctor could turn a breech baby, deliver a difficult presentation, mend a serious tear, and use forceps skillfully when necessary. But contemporary physicians know very little about how to manage a normal delivery. In most medical centers, residents are taught how to perform general, rather than local, anesthesia. In fact, many physicians have stated that they simply *don't know* how to do breech vaginals anymore.

Cohen and Estner quote one obstetrician as saying:

> Recently I had two breeches close together, assisted at each delivery by a first- or second-year resident. I discovered that these fellows knew practically nothing about breech delivery. They assumed that every breech was going to be delivered by cesarean section, and when it came to the delivery, they knew nothing about getting the arms out, about delivering the after-coming head, the use of Piper forceps, or any such things.

The authors note that many institutions now deliver 60 to 90 percent of their breech presentations surgically, yet there has not been a measurable improvement in infant outcome.

One justification for performing excessive cesareans is the threat of mal-

*Written in collaboration with Cathrin Prince Leslie, midwife.

practice suits. If the baby is born "less than perfect," the obstetrician can say that he or she did everything that could be done. This is an unfortunate state of affairs, and we're going to have to work with doctors to find a reasonable solution to this problem if we hope to change childbirth practices.

Cesarean Delivery

When nature is allowed to take her course, babies are massaged and hugged into the world by their mother's bodies. The baby's nervous system uses the tactile stimulation to activate its principal organ systems. Normal labor contractions increase the production of lecithin in the air sacs of the baby's lungs, which prepares them to function after birth. As the baby descends through the birth canal, the lung fluid is squeezed out of the air sacs, enabling adequate aeration of the lungs.

When a baby is born by cesarean, you have to wait while you're being sutured before you can hold your baby in your arms. It's less rewarding to gaze into your baby's eyes when you and your baby are groggy and irritable from the anesthesia. And then, you may have pain from the operation. It's hard to move your body after surgery, making it difficult to breastfeed. And there may be numbness in your breasts, which deprive you of some of the pleasurable sensations of the first hours with your newborn. Some 30 percent of cesarean babies are taken to intensive care, where they remain in the hospital about three times as long, depriving them of the vital bonding process with their parent(s).

Many mothers experience guilt, anger, depression, and feelings of helplessness after a cesarean. Then they feel guilty that they aren't simply grateful because they have a whole and (perhaps) healthy baby. They grieve for their femininity and for a feeling of trust and confidence in their bodies. They blame themselves and do not "feel like a mother" until about a month later than vaginally delivered women. And that first month is crucial to the bonding process.

Presumably, the main justification for having a cesarean is to save the baby's life, and rarely, to save the mother's life. And yet, the mortality rate is four times higher for babies delivered surgically than for infants delivered vaginally. It could be argued that primarily high-risk babies would be delivered by cesarean, and yet statistics show that in some cases, even very high-risk mothers have a lower rate of infant death when babies are born at home where, obviously, they will be delivered vaginally.

Cesarean babies have an overall rate of illness that is ten times higher than vaginally delivered babies. This is partly because of the drugs administered to the mother during the cesarean, which pass through the placenta, and the drugs given to the mother for pain after the cesarean, which pass through the breast milk.

If a cesarean is being performed because the woman is believed to be overdue, there is a danger that the dates were misjudged, and the baby may be delivered prematurely. Then the baby's lungs may be too immature to bring enough oxygen to its body, resulting in respiratory distress syndrome. This is one reason why premature babies who are delivered surgically are seven times more likely to die than vaginally delivered babies. Premature babies and others who do not have the opportunity to bond with their parents are more likely to become battered children, according to a study reported by M. Lynch in *Lancet*.

For the mother, cesarean section carries the same risks as all major surgery. The average blood loss is about twice that of normal birth. Studies from California, Georgia, and Rhode Island indicate that there are from two to twenty-six times more maternal deaths from cesareans than from vaginal deliveries. These studies indicate that most risks are due to the anesthesia and the surgery rather than any condition that led the physician to choose to perform the cesarean.

Furthermore, death by cesarean is under-reported, because it is reported as death due to surgery, or to pulmonary embolism, or complications of anesthesia. When women die from complications that occur after the operation, the cause of death is not given as the cesarean.

The National Institute of Child Health and Human Development (NIH) Task Force determined that "cesarean delivery carries about four times the risk of maternal mortality of a vaginal delivery" and that maternal morbidity (disease) rates are generally five to ten times higher after cesarean delivery than after vaginal delivery.

When Is a Cesarean Needed?

Helen Marieskind, author of *An Evaluation of Cesarean Section in the United States*, divides the indications for cesarean section into two categories: absolute indications and relative indications. In between these are gray area indications, which have to be evaluated on an individual basis.

Absolute Indications

In these circumstances, no other method of delivery is likely to produce a healthy, live baby.

Maternal Pelvic Contraction. In this case the pelvis cannot accommodate a mature fetus, possibly due to an injury or extreme malnutrition. This is a rare condition.

Prolapsed Umbilical Cord. When the cord precedes the baby in the birth canal, the baby's head presses down upon the cord and can cut off its blood and oxygen, causing injury or death. This is often an iatrogenic (physician-caused) problem, since premature rupture of the bag of waters (to speed up delivery) can result in a prolapsed cord.

Placenta Previa. When the entire placenta implants over the opening of the cervix, normal delivery is impossible.

Placenta Abruptio. When the placenta separates from the uterine wall before the birth of the baby, it can cause dangerous hemorrhaging.

Transverse Presentation. When the baby cannot be moved to a more favorable position for delivery, a cesarean is necessary.

Gray Areas

These conditions can be dangerous, but they vary according to individual circumstances.

Diabetes. In the past, babies of diabetic mothers often died when pregnancy went beyond thirty-eight weeks, so cesareans were performed routinely. Modern medical advances in the care of the pregnant diabetic mother are now allowing some diabetic women to carry to term and delivery vaginally.

Heart Disease. Women with heart disease are usually delivered by cesarean, but medical advances are enabling some of these women to deliver vaginally.

Active Herpes Sores. Women with active herpes lesions were formerly delivered by cesarean, but now some of these babies can be delivered safely, depending on the location of the sores.

Blood Incompatibility. Cesareans used to be necessary if the mother had RH-negative blood and the baby had RH-positive blood. Now there are new methods of preventing maternal sensitization. But if the fetus is endangered by anemia as a result of RH disease and the delivery cannot be induced safely and successfully, a cesarean is required.

Toxemia. When toxemia becomes life-threatening, and induction has been attempted without success, a cesarean is probably necessary.

Relative Indications

The following conditions can usually be avoided by finding a patient, noninterventionist care giver.

Dystocia (Prolonged Labor). This catch-all term is responsible for 30 percent of the increased cesarean rates. It includes cephalopelvic disproportion, fetopelvic disproportion, and "labor dysfunction."
CPD (cephalopelvic disproportion) is the indicated when the baby's head is considered too large to pass through the mother's pelvis. This is the pri-

mary cause of cesarean sections. In fetopelvic disproportion the whole baby is considered too large to pass through the mother's pelvis. Labor dysfunction includes such terms as "failure to progress," "prolonged labor," and "uterine inertia."

All of the above must be regarded with extreme caution. It's improbable that North American women's pelvises are getting smaller. It's far more likely that the nervousness of obstetricians, their lack of training in the art of obstetrics, the tight schedules of hospitals, and the general lack of support for the normally laboring woman is at fault. Dystocia is primarily an iatrogenic (doctor-caused) problem. Keeping women on their backs instead of allowing gravity to aid in childbirth is a major hazard with dystocia. The squatting position increases the size of the pelvis by more than a centimeter. The very threat of possibly having to have a cesarean undoubtedly contributes to dystocia.

At The Farm community in Tennessee, 1,200 births were performed over a period of ten years, and 98.1 percent were entirely without interventions. Ina May Gaskin, their first midwife, tells women that neither the pelvis nor the baby's head is a fixed size. Even if the pelvis is small, a fine natural delivery is still possible, provided the mother is strong and patient, "the rushes strong, and the vibrations good."

"Failure to progress" is another catch-all term which simply means that the woman's labor is not going as fast as her doctor wants it to go. Most midwives will allow a woman to labor at her own pace, whatever that may be. Ina May Gaskin says, "You don't have to have any preconceived notions about what is too long for the first stage. If the mother is replenishing her energy by eating and sleeping, rushes are light, the baby's head is not being tightly squeezed and the membranes are still intact, the first stage can stretch over three or four days and still be perfectly normal."

Cesareans are obviously not intended to protect the mother, because the maternal mortality rate for cesareans is 41.9 deaths per 100,000, as compared with 11.1 deaths per 100,000 vaginal deliveries.

Fetal Distress. While there is no evidence that the actual incidence of fetal distress has changed, the diagnosis of fetal distress has become much more common over the past ten years. This condition arises from inadequate fetal oxygen supply and carbon dioxide removal.

This is another case of iatrogenic problems. Keeping a woman flat on her back, using pitocin to speed up contractions, and using the electronic fetal monitor have all contributed to a higher incidence of this diagnosis, leading to an increase in cesareans. Many infants who were in distress according to the monitor were found to be healthy at birth.

Failed Induction. One method of inducing labor is to artificially rupture the membranes (the bag of waters). This method has a high failure rate. Because there is believed to be an increased susceptibility to infection after a prolonged period of time, a cesarean is often performed. That "prolonged period" used to be seventy-two hours, but now it may be twelve hours. Before subjecting yourself to a cesarean, you should know that the rate of infections with cesareans is extremely high, and so it is a dubious way of preventing infection. And this is, of course, yet another good reason not to rupture the membranes in the first place, unless it is absolutely necessary.

Cohen and Estner suggest that if your doctor wants to perform a cesarean because of "prolonged rupture of the membranes," you can get a reading on your blood pressure and your temperature. If neither is high, it is unlikely that infection is present.

Prematurity, Low Birth Weight. Undersized babies are believed to be too fragile to tolerate normal labor. Since cesareans have become popular, there have been improved survival rates for these infants. However, the use of diagnostic ultrasound has led to a frequent misdiagnosis of prematurity, and infants delivered by cesarean who are not actually premature are at greater risk than they would have been if delivered vaginally. A midwife or doctor with sensitive hands can learn to feel for the size of a baby in utero. If the art of obstetrics is revived, we may be able to reserve this use of cesarean delivery for those cases when it is genuinely necessary.

Previous Cesarean Delivery. Ninety-eight percent of mothers in the United States who delivered a previous baby by cesarean are having repeat surgical deliveries. This accounts for over 30 percent of the cesareans being performed. In most cases, *this is absolutely unnecessary.*

Vaginal Birth After Cesarean (VBAC)

Vaginal birth after cesarean (VBAC) is the norm in almost every country in the world, apart from the United States and Canada.

During a cesarean, two incisions are made. The first cut goes through the abdomen. The "bikini cut" or "smile" is the most common abdominal cut. It is made horizontally just below the pubic hairline. A less common abdominal cut is sometimes made vertically from the navel to the pubis. The abdominal cut is the one you see.

The second cut, the uterine incision, is the one that affects your future attempts to deliver a baby vaginally. The most common uterine incision is the lower segment horizontal (or transverse) incision. This cut is excellent for VBACs because it cuts the uterus at the bottom, in the segment that does the least amount of work during labor.

Back in 1916, a physician coined the phrase, "Once a cesarean, always a cesarean." At that time the classical cut, which extended from the middle of the uterus to the top, cutting through the part that contracts most energetically during labor, was used. In 1916, the maternal mortality rate for cesareans was at least ten percent. Women who had previous cesareans were not allowed to go into labor because maternal mortality rose toward thirty percent if there had been an attempt at vaginal delivery, especially if several vaginal exams were performed.

This high mortality rate resulted from poor suturing materials, unsterile conditions, and difficulties with anesthesia. There were no blood banks nor antibiotics. Under such dire circumstances, combined with the disadvantage of the classical incision, physicians rightfully determined that subsequent pregnancies were safer when performed as repeat cesareans, which would be scheduled before the woman was due to go into labor.

In the 1930s the transverse cut became popular. It became safe to perform cesareans, even late in labor. The transverse cut greatly diminished the chances of massive hemorrhage, and it healed more rapidly. It became reasonable to consider a trial of labor and vaginal birth after cesarean.

When the advantages of the transverse cut are combined with sterile procedures, good suturing materials and techniques, access to excellent blood transfusion services, blood volume expanders, and antibiotics, a trial by labor and a possible vaginal birth are actually *safer* than an automatic repeat cesarean.

When you combine these factors with plenty of patience and support for the laboring woman and a minimum number of vaginal exams, you have an excellent chance of having a vaginal birth after a cesarean.

Yet most physicians and patients still believe that there is a terrible danger of uterine rupture when a woman attempts to deliver vaginally after having had a cesarean. Women are threatened with the specter of permanent sterility if they are irresponsible enough to consider this option.

Rupture is a very rare occurrence. Cohen and Estner surveyed the literature on recent American obstetrical articles and found "*no instances of catastrophic lower segment uterine rupture*. Several articles had no incidences of uterine rupture. In the infrequent references to 'uterine rupture,' rupture was generally benign."

In fact, rupture is far more common in a non-cesarean uterus. The harsh contractions caused by inducing labor with pitocin put a great strain on the uterus. And yet one doesn't hear of physicians advising against induction because of the danger of a ruptured uterus.

In *Silent Knife*, Cohen and Estner elaborate:

A 1980 study by Golan reported 93 cases of uterine rupture during a five-year period. Sixty-one ruptures occurred in normal uteri, while thirty-two were found in women who had had a previous cesarean. There were nine maternal deaths, *all in the group of women who had not previously had cesarean surgery*. In the rare circumstance that a uterus with a previous cesarean does separate, the incision generally opens gently and neatly, like a seam or a zipper. *We*

found no reports of maternal death associated with the lower seg-
ment incision in all the studies we surveyed; the incidence of fetal
death associated with VBAC is agreed to be less than that with elec-
tive repeat cesarean even by the most reluctant VBAC skeptics.

In fact, it has been shown that a well-healed scar is as strong as the uterus itself. The area of the incision is more resistant to rupture under tension
than other portions of the uterus. Physicians often cannot find the original
incision because the wound has healed so well. And even if the scar does separate, there is no pain.

The dangers inherent in any cesarean delivery (which are grossly *under*emphasized) are far greater than the potential danger of a vaginal delivery
after a cesarean. A study done in 1981 on repeat cesareans stated that allowing a trial of labor resulted in thirty-seven *fewer* infant deaths and 0.7 fewer
maternal deaths per 10,000 pregnant women.

So—can a "ruptured" uterus lead to permanent sterility? In a study of
526 women by Merrill and Gibbs, they found a 0.5 percent rate of "rupture."
Of these, there was no hemorrhage or shock, and only 1 hysterectomy was
performed.

If you are considering a VBAC, please read *Silent Knife* by Nancy Wainer Cohen and Lois J. Estner and study the current literature on the subject.

Cesarean Prevention

If you are advised that you will need a cesarean before you go into labor, get
a second opinion from a physician who has been recommended by someone
other than your present doctor. A knowledgeable midwife should be able to
refer you to a reliable doctor. Otherwise, contact private prenatal teachers,
women's health collectives, and so on.

There are several ways to avoid unnecessary cesareans. First, hire a midwife or labor coach who is well-informed and who can help you make a decision that will feel good to you. Find someone who works in collaboration
with physicians. She or he should have skills to advise you during pregnancy
and birth regarding healthy procedures and how to avoid unnecessary interventions. This person should be able to detect variations from normal and
to inform you of your choices. If you do go to a hospital, your midwife or
labor coach should be able to go with you and stay until the baby is born.

Births that are planned to take place at home have a much lower cesarean rate. If a home birth isn't right for you, staying at home until your labor
is *well* advanced (six centimeters or more of dilation) is a good safeguard.
You'll need an experienced midwife or birth attendant to advise you on this.

Be in touch with your body, your feelings, your senses. While you are
pregnant you can massage your body and have others massage it for you.
You can keep your emotions clear by facing your feelings—both positive and
negative. You can talk about your fears with your midwife, your partner,

your friends. You can honor your intuition by paying attention to your cravings for various foods (within reason).

While you're in labor, be conscious of the signals you receive from your body. If you're in tune with your body, you'll know when to eat, when to walk, when to breathe deeply, and when to push. It also helps to stroke your belly and communicate with your baby, because you'll need to work together when you're in labor.

Try to find a physician who is able to listen to your needs and who respects your ability to birth your baby and make intelligent decisions for yourself and your family. Does this doctor intend to deliver your baby for you, or will he or she lend support for you to deliver your own baby? What is this doctor's rate of cesareans? (Your local midwives will know which doctors are the least interventionist.)

If You Must Have A Cesarean

If a cesarean is unavoidable for yourself or your baby's safety, these suggestions will help you to make it a better experience.

- Find out the protocol at the hospital where your doctor has privileges. If you're unhappy with any of their routines, protest before you have the baby.
- In most cases, it's better to go into labor before a cesarean.
- There is no need for prophylactic I.V. if there is to be a transverse cut, since it will not cause massive hemorrhage.
- Epidural anesthesia has the lowest rate of side effects and allows you to be conscious so that you can see and touch your baby immediately. It does, however, take a more skilled anesthetist to administer it.
- Many hospitals now allow the father and birth attendant to be with you during a cesarean when epidural or spinal anesthesia are used. Neither you nor the father will actually see the surgery (you'll be draped) but you'll be there to greet your little one. If the baby is well, he or she is usually wrapped and given to the father to hold. Your baby can be held close to you while you're being sutured.
- Dr. Marshall Klaus suggests that about twenty minutes after the birth, mother, infant, and father go to a room where they have privacy. The infant can be placed next to the mother with a heat panel. Here the mother can have the normal forty-five to sixty minutes together with her newborn and her partner. Every ten to fifteen minutes the pulse rate and blood pressure will be taken, but otherwise you should not be interrupted. During this period your anesthesia continues, so you are free to explore and enjoy your new infant.
- If your baby must go to the nursery, see if the father can go along.
- If you must be separated from your baby, try to minimize the time you spend apart. Mentally, send your love to your baby. Since pink is the

color of love, imagine sending pink light. Reach out with your heart and embrace your baby in spirit. Create an imaginary sanctuary space where the two of you can meet and enjoy one another. Once you are reunited, take the time to heal the separation. Speak to your baby and tell him or her how much you missed being together. This could be a healing process that will be repeated when your child is actually old enough to respond to you. Cohen and Estner tell of an incident where the mother described her feelings about the birth to her eight-year-old daughter, and the child responded by saying, "Mommy, I missed you at that time, too, and I was happy when you took care of me all by yourself!"

- Give yourself permission to feel all of your feelings for at least the next year. You may want to allow yourself to grieve about the loss of the kind of delivery you hoped to have. You may need to review exactly what happened and your feelings may include anger, sadness, powerlessness, loss of autonomy, loss of control, lowered self-esteem, guilt, and many others. If you can express your feelings, no matter how irrational they seem, it will eventually make you feel better, and it will improve your chances of having a more positive relationship with your child and a better birth experience next time. Your local cesarean birth group or postpartum group may be able to offer direct support, or they may refer you to someone who can help you.

REFERENCES

Yvonne Brackbill, Ph.D., June Rice, and Diony Young, *Birth Trap* (Warner Books, 1984).

Nancy Wainer Cohen and Lois J. Estner, *Silent Knife* (Bergin & Garvey Publishers. Inc., 1983).

Neal Devitt, "The Transition from Home to Hospital Birth in the United States, 1930-1960," *Birth and the Family Journal* 4, 1977.

Kirsten Emmott, M.D., Statement on Midwifery and Home Birth (Vancouver, B.C., 1986).

Ina May Gaskin, *Spiritual Midwifery* (The Book Publishing Co., 1977).

Doris Haire, "Fetal Effects of Ultrasound, A Growing Controversy," *Journal of Nurse-Midwifery*, 29, No. 4, (July/August) 1984.

Elizabeth B. Harvey, et al, "Prenatal X-Ray Exposure and Childhood Cancer in Twins," *The New England Journal of Medicine*, 312, No. 9, (February), 1985.

Robert A. Hatcher, M.D., et al, *Contraceptive Technology, 1976-1977* (Irvington Publishers, 1976).

Marshall H. Klaus, et al, *Bonding, The Beginnings of Parent-Infant Attachment* (C.V. Mosby Company, 1983).

W. R. Lee, "Working with Visual Display Units," *British Medical Journal*, October 1985.

Doreen Liebeskind, M.D. et al, "Diagnostic Ultrasound: Effects on the DNA and Growth Patterns of Animal Cells," *Radiology*, 131, (April) 1979.

Helen Marieskind, *An Evaluation of Cesarean Section in the United States* (Department of Health, Education and Welfare, 1979).

Lewis Mehl, M.D. et al, "Evaluation of Outcomes of Non-nurse Midwives: Matched Comparisons with Physicians," *Women and Health*, 4, 1980.

Lewis Mehl, M.D., et al, "Home Birth Versus Hospital Birth: Comparisons of Outcomes of Matched Populations," *Pregnancy, Childbirth, and Parenthood*, edited by Paul Ahmed (Elsevier, 1981).

National Institutes of Child Health and Human Development, "Draft Report of the Task Force on Cesarean Childbirth," NIH, (September)1980.

D. J. Pizzarello et al, "Effect of Pulsed Low-Power Ultrasound on Growing Tissues, II: Malignant Tissues," *Exp. Cell Biology*, 46, (April) 1978.

Stanley Sagov et al, *Home Birth, A Practitioner's Guide to Birth Outside the Hospital* (Aspen, 1984).

Madeleine Shearer, "Complications of Cesarean to Mother and Infant," *Birth and Family Journal*, 4, No. 3, (Fall) 1977.

M. E. Stratmeyer, Ph.D., "Research in Ultrasound Bioeffects: A Public Health View," *Birth and the Family Journal*, 7, No. 2, (Summer) 1980.

Marjorie Tew, "Place of Birth and Perintal Mortality," *Journal of the Royal College of General Practitioners*, 35, 1985.

Chapter 5
LABOR AND BIRTH

When I had my first baby in 1966, the Lamaze breathing technique was becoming popular. Birth classes were starting up, and couples were being trained in rigorous Pavlovian responses to the three stages of labor. The Lamaze technique attempts to prevent pain by deliberately distracting the woman's attention from what is happening within her body.

At first I was offended by the idea of being trained to pant like a Pavlovian dog and respond in a predictable way to each stage of labor. But since I wanted a natural birth and I was afraid of being in pain, I learned the Lamaze technique. And it served me well—under the circumstances.

I couldn't find a midwife in New York City in 1966. But I stayed at home as long as possible. My waters broke and I had mild contractions for twenty-four hours. I called the hospital and spoke to a doctor who insisted that I come in, because he said there was a danger of infection. At the hospital, they told me that my baby would be in danger if I labored too long, so they would have to induce labor. They gave me pitocin, which caused intense and painful contractions. I was expected to deliver flat on my back, with an I.V. in my arm. Approximately once an hour the obstetrician came in to do a painful internal exam. I was given very little encouragement to birth naturally, and the obstetrician repeatedly expressed his opinion that I should be delivered by cesarean—which I resisted.

Under these adverse circumstances, Lamaze breathing served me well. It was well-suited to the mechanistic, sterile environment in which I was expected to perform the most sensual, the most feminine, the most vulnerable act of my entire life. Lamaze gave me the armoring that I needed.

But during the last ten years, there's been a shift away from Lamaze training. Since every birth is unique, many contemporary midwives and childbirth educators counsel that the best way to prepare for labor is to get in tune with yourself, your body, your baby, and to have good communication with your midwife and your partner.

In this concept of childbirth, the baby takes on a significant role. Dr. Verny's book, *The Secret Life of the Unborn Child*, and similar studies have made us aware that the baby is an alert participant in the birthing process.

And finally, the midwife or labor coach plays an essential role. Even a well-meaning doctor rarely has the time to sit with you throughout your labor. Regardless of whether you have your baby at home or in a hospital, the most important thing for your sense of security and well-being throughout labor is to have someone constantly with you whom you can rely on, who is experienced and empathetic, who cares about you, and who will put your needs first at all times. This will enable you to relax and to be in tune with your body, which will enhance your chances of having a natural birth.

We attach so much importance to the short period of time when we labor and deliver our baby because it is the prelude to the magical moment of birth — it is like falling in love and getting married at the same time.

No wonder we put so much energy into preparing for it. No wonder we want everything to be perfect. No wonder we want a bridesmaid to be with us every step of the way, sharing our joys, our sorrows, our apprehensions. No wonder we want our lover to be there, too. No wonder we want to be in a pleasant environment, surrounded by kind people.

And yet, the wedding is only a moment. And the rest of the marriage does not necessarily depend on how the wedding goes. So if the moment of birth is disappointing, it is never too late to embrace your little one and hold this child in your arms and look into his or her eyes, and allow the love to flow between you.

BREATHING*

Graduated breathing techniques, as taught in many prenatal classes are distraction techniques that can be exhausting. Many women find themselves frustrated because they relied on techniques to disguise or avoid the power of labor and they missed out on the experience of actually giving birth. These techniques remove the woman's attention from her body and her baby. Having to stay in control causes her to tighten both her jaw and her pelvis, which prevents her from being flexible, from bending, from turning, from being attuned to the ever-changing needs of her body.

As Elizabeth Noble says in *Childbirth With Insight*, "Most childbirth preparation promises a control that can never be realized because of the nature of birth . . . the harder we try to fall asleep, to remember a name, to have an orgasm, or to become pregnant, the more it seems to escape us. Yet when we give up, what we seek may happen easily." Noble quotes from Erich Fromm: "Every act of birth requires the courage to let go of something . . . to let go eventually of all certainties, and to rely on one thing: one's own power to be aware and to respond; that is, one's creativity."

Breathing from the chest, as taught in Lamaze classes, uses the muscles of the shoulder and neck. It requires lifting the whole thoracic cavity: heart, lungs, and rib cage. People tend to breathe this way when they are very anxious or tense. On the other hand, breathing from the diaphragm uses only one muscle, the diaphragm. It centers the attention at the solar plexus, just

*Written in collaboration with Cathrin Prince Leslie, midwife.

above the womb, which is your center of power. And it expands the womb, allowing plenty of space for the baby to move and the contractions to take place.

Breathing is something everyone does. Our bodies know how to breathe. We never have to remind our lungs to do it. Breath is life-sustaining power. During labor, we dance the dance which brings new life into this world. Connecting with our breath helps us to connect with ourselves and with the process of giving birth. Our breath forms the rhythm and the contractions form the beat as we dance the dance of life, the dance of birth.

While you are pregnant, be aware of your breathing. Take time to consciously relax. Tune into your center with your breath. Breathe out the tension from each area of your body, releasing as you exhale. Remember that labor is a releasing — an opening up and letting go.

When you get into a situation of anxiety that causes you to tighten up, your breathing usually changes. Use your releasing breaths to bring you back to center — back to calmness. You can become aware of your breathing and use it more consciously in your day-to-day life.

When you find yourself feeling tense, observe your breath. You'll probably find that you're holding your breath or breathing in a very shallow way. Of course, holding your breath deprives you of oxygen, and just increases your tension. Try taking a deep breath, and as you exhale, make a sound like "heh" or "hoh" from deep in your chest, and hold it for the length of the exhalation.

Now inhale and exhale again, making the sound, and think of the vibrations of that sound moving to any part of your body where you are holding tension. Inhale and exhale again, making the deep sound, and feel your breath and the sound carrying away any possible tension, anger, or tightness.

Now inhale and feel how good it is to take in a fresh breath of air. Then exhale, and make a deep sound and think of the vibration of that sound moving through your womb, through your cervix, and out your vagina, opening and releasing and making way for your baby.

During labor, remember that instead of holding your breath and trying to block out the pain, tune into the pain, inhale deeply, and as you exhale, make a sound that expresses what you are feeling: moan, groan, sigh, wail, or scream. Allow yourself to become primitive and animalistic.

Giving birth is a sensual experience. One of the midwives at The Farm community in Tennessee said, "Over and over again, I've seen that the best way to get a baby out is by cuddling and smooching with your husband. That loving, sexy vibe is what puts the baby in there, and it's what gets it out, too." And Sufi Master Hazrat Inayat Khan said, "With love, even the rocks will open." (These are quotes from *Spiritual Midwifery* by Ina May Gaskin.)

As her labor progresses, a woman who is encouraged to express herself freely may make sounds similar to having a prolonged orgasm. During delivery she may scream in pain or in rapture. These sounds help to open and relax her pelvis and her cervix. Yet there are few places where such "uncivilized" noises are encouraged. A supportive attendant can encourage such behavior. The mother can discuss her fears openly. She can cry or scream or do whatever she needs to do without fear of being judged.

Many people are shy about using their voice forcefully, so practice using your voice whenever you get a chance. Sing along with the songs on the stereo. When you're in the shower, sing out at the top of your lungs. You'll find it feels good, and you may even get a few laughs!

Though it may sound a bit peculiar, another way to convince yourself of the power of your voice is to rehearse while having a bowel movement. Ideally, one should be patient and relaxed during a bowel movement, but for the sake of this exercise, try pushing while holding your breath. Then try pushing while making a deep sound. You will probably find that the latter is much more effective.

Besides your breathing, remember to tune in to your baby. This is a labor that both of you will be doing together. If you are in harmony with each other, the labor is more likely to go smoothly.

For more information, please see Recommended Books, particularly *Childbirth With Insight* and *Birthing Normally*.

POSITIONS FOR BIRTHING

At a Midwifery Conference in Vancouver, B.C. in 1986, I saw a slide show presented by Janet Issac Ashford of artwork on the theme of women giving birth throughout history. She showed one slide after another of women giving birth, in a variety of cultures, in a variety of positions: standing, leaning, and squatting. Usually these women were surrounded by loving, empathetic companions—mostly women. Their faces showed expressions of intense but bearable pain, of rapture, and of victory.

These beautiful dramatic settings were in sharp contrast with the pictures that began to occur in the mid-1800s, when men began to take over the birth process. Suddenly women made to lie down and become passive victims ("patients") in a process where men were increasingly the "doers," and the women's midwives and companions were replaced mostly by machines.

Dr. Michel Odent is a non-interventionist physician who has become famous for his maternity unit in Pithiviers, France. He encourages each woman to find the position for birthing in which she feels most comfortable. He has observed that most mothers walk around during labor until the end of the first stage. Then they often choose a hands-and-knees position. At the time of birth, they may squat while supported by their husband and midwife. However, he does not ask a woman to follow any set of rules. He encourages her to tune in to her own body, and respond to its signals from her own center.

For more information, please see the Recommended Books, particularly *Active Birth* and *Birth Reborn*.

USING YOUR INTUITION

We're entering an age in which the rational mind no longer needs to be in complete control. We're learning that our intuitive minds have a unique intelligence of their own, a female intelligence, an inner knowingness that cannot be explained. And we are learning that when we dare to follow this inner knowingness, we are almost always right.

But the rational mind is threatened by having to share its power. And the rational mind is very clever. It turns us against the intuitive mind by making lots of noise whenever the intuitive mind makes a mistake. In fact, it makes so much noise that we forget to notice the myriad of mistakes that the rational mind makes.

If you were to make a chart of all the times that you had an intuitive insight or hunch or feeling — and if you made notes on what happened when you did or didn't follow your intuition, you would find (if you are like most people) that nine out of ten times, when you followed your intuition, you were glad you had.

But your rational mind would take the one time that you were wrong, and never let you forget it. In this way, your confidence in your intuitive mind would be undermined. And you would ignore the fact that the rational mind does very well if it is right nine out of ten times.

Most midwives follow their intuition, and they encourage their women clients to do the same. It is a happy combination, with glowing results.

TUNING IN ON YOUR BABY

We pay so much attention to our labor that we tend to forget about the baby, who is experiencing the most intense time of its life. If you remember to be conscious of your baby and of the inner workings of your own body, I believe your labor will proceed more smoothly.

I was present at a birth where the mother was tired and feeling overwhelmed by laboring for so long. I urged her to breathe deeply, to relax, to turn inward and concentrate on her baby. To welcome her baby. To stroke it and speak to it. To think of her womb and her birth canal and her baby working together, creating birth together.

Soon she was stroking her belly, saying repeatedly, encouragingly, gently, "Come on, baby. Come on, baby." Then she felt a new confidence, a surge of strength, and the baby was born soon after.

Have you ever wondered how being born feels to the baby? Through hypnosis, I've helped many people to re-live their time in the womb and their birth experiences. Here are a couple of examples.

RHODA: I'm suspended in space. My body can fold in half, and I'm looking between my legs. I feel a constriction in my heart; a feeling of pressure.

(Silence.) I'm getting bigger. I can see my hands. I feel hair growing on my head. There's light in here. I want to look around, but I can't turn my own head. There's a tight feeling in my heart.

I feel a kind of dread. I don't think my mother will be able to relate to me. I'm not sure I want to be born. I'm afraid of meeting my mother.

(Silence.) Now I'm being delivered, and my mother is asleep. Different women are handling me. Now I'm being cleaned. The woman is rough, and she handles me as if I didn't have any feelings. As if I wasn't a person. I'm being passed from one woman to another.

This one is nice. She whispers to me, "You're pretty!"

* * *

JOANNIE: I feel like I'm sliding out against my will — like gravity is pulling me down. I feel sad that I'm leaving. I want my Mom to reassure me that she'll help me to leave and that she'll be there when I arrive in the world. But I don't get that from her. She loves me. But she's very scared. She's not concentrating on me. The pressure is on my head — really strong.

(Silence.) My eyes are hurting. They put something in my eyes. I've been born, and I'm glad about that. I'm glad to be here. I feel wanted. I feel loved. I'm being held in my mother's arms. She's so loving. I'm being nursed. I feel warm. There's a lot of love here. My Dad is looking at me and he's proud of me; he thinks I'm really something!

HAVING A BIRTH ATTENDANT

Studies in Guatemala showed that women who had birth attendants, when compared with those who did not, were in labor for approximately half as long! And after the birth, these women stayed awake longer and stroked their babies and smiled and talked to their babies more than the control group.

How could this be? Dr. Marshall Klaus, who conducted the study, suggested that when a woman is anxious, her adrenalin level shoots up which affects the uterine muscle by decreasing contractions.

Another doctor and researcher, O'Driscoll, applies this concept to eight thousand patients per year at the Rotunda in Dublin. He provides a personal nurse to stay with every mother throughout labor. He found that this so shortened the duration of labor that no increase in nursing staff was required to provide this additional attention to birthing women.

In France, Dr. Michel Odent says that particularly with a high-risk labor it is important to avoid the physiological disturbances induced by a conventional hospital atmosphere — unless it has become apparent that a cesarean cannot be avoided.

Odent provides women with a homelike atmosphere, semidarkness, silence, a caring midwife, and vertical postures. He says this helps her to reach a level of consciousness that is on a par with reduced adrenergic secretion and an optimum natural secretion of oxytocin and probably of endorphins. This natural body chemistry gives energy, intensifies contractions, and helps the woman to feel more relaxed and less sensitive to pain.

Out of 150 societies studied by anthropologists, all but one had the tradition of a family member or friend staying with the mother during labor and birth.

HOW TO RECOGNIZE LABOR

Labor is not always self-evident. Other bodily processes can mimic the contractions of labor: urinary tract infections, dysentery, and the griping caused by laxatives. The latter two can set off the real contractions of labor.

How can you distinguish false contractions from real labor? Real labor tends to start out mildly; contractions may be about fifteen minutes apart and fifteen seconds long. Real labor tends to get stronger gradually and progressively. Real labor will usually get stronger if you get up and walk around. On the other hand, false labor may start strong and suddenly, with contractions five minutes apart and one minute long. If you get up and walk around, these contractions will usually slack off.

STAGES OF LABOR

The first stage of labor begins when the uterine muscles contract at regular intervals and get increasingly stronger. The womb or uterus looks like a pear, with the narrow end or neck at the bottom. The cervix is the neck of the womb. At the bottom of the cervix is a small opening, which is the mouth of the uterus. The mouth is about the size of the opening of a man's penis. This mouth of the uterus is usually sealed by mucus, which prevents foreign matter from entering the womb.

At the beginning of labor, there may be a bloody show when the mucus plug in the cervix comes out and there is a release of blood and mucus. The first stage continues while the baby descends down the birth canal, its head pushing against the cervix.

As the baby's head pushes against this opening, the tissue of the cervix thins out (like a balloon, as it is blown up), and the opening gets miraculously bigger and bigger. This is called dilation, and it is measured by centimeters. Each centimeter is about the width of a finger. The first stage may take from twelve to fifteen hours with the first baby, and less with later babies, but every woman is different.

When the cervix is fully dilated at about ten centimeters, it is large enough for a baby's head to pass through, and you have reached the stage of transition, or the second stage of labor.

The second stage may last from a few minutes up to three hours of more. You will feel an almost uncontrollable urge to push. Your midwife or doctor will tell you when to push so that you are less likely to tear as the baby spontaneously turns ninety degrees and comes out into the world.

When the baby is born, you have reached the third stage of labor. The cord may be cut and you may be completely relaxed and nursing your baby (which stimulates contractions) when your uterus contracts again — after about ten to twenty minutes — and the placenta or "afterbirth" comes out. This is usually a painless procedure.

DURING LABOR

Nourishment During Labor

Labor does not slow digestion. If you desire food, some doctors now recommend that you eat a nutritious meal just after you go into labor, because if you have a long labor without nourishment, you're likely to feel too weak to continue without help. After this initial (optional) meal, solid foods are usually avoided.

When I went into labor with my first baby, I had a strong craving for a baked potato with sour cream. Contrary to all rules, I followed my intuition. I can't imagine how I could have gotten through thirty-six hours of labor without that extra boost of carbohydrates and protein.

By the way, the father should be sure to eat, too, because a hungry father is an impatient father, and impatience is to easily communicated to the laboring mother. The same is true for the midwife and other assistants.

It's essential to keep your blood sugar up during labor because if your blood sugar gets too low, you'll feel tired and depressed and your uterus won't contract as well during or after the delivery — which increases the possibility of hemorrhage.

Here are some good forms of nourishment during labor, and most of them will also help maintain your blood sugar level.

Warm Milk With Honey. This is relaxing because of its high calcium content, and it provides a quick blood sugar boost and protein and fats to maintain the blood sugar level. (Try warm soy milk with honey if you're allergic to cow's milk.)

Miso Broth. Made from a high-protein soybean paste, miso is very nourishing and strengthening and easy to prepare. It is available from most health food stores.

Miso Broth. Boil 1 cup of water. Put 1 tablespoon miso in a cup, and add a couple of tablespoons of boiling water. Stir until it makes a kind of paste, and then gradually add the rest of the water while stirring. Drink as often as you like.

Blue Cohosh, Squaw Vine, Raspberry Leaf, and Peppermint Tea with Honey. Any of these teas, taken separately or together, are perfect for labor.

Tea with honey and lemon can be frozen into little ice cubes to suck on during labor. This will help keep your mouth moist during the heavy breathing of labor. If you only have large cubes, you can put a few in a clean towel or cloth, and hammer them into chips.

If you don't like blue cohosh (which has a strong taste and smell), you can substitute spikenard. This herb is favored by some women as a good aid to childbirth.

Blue Cohosh, Squaw Vine, Raspberry Leaf, and Peppermint Tea. Boil 2 cups water. Add ½ teaspoon of each herb. Brew in a covered pot for 15 minutes. Be sure to add plenty of honey, (preferably raw) to keep the blood sugar high. Add lemon if you like, too.

Ginger Tea. This tea is stimulating and soothing. You can drink one or two cups during a day of labor.

Ginger Tea. Add 1 teaspoon dried ginger pieces or 2 teaspoons freshly grated ginger to 1 cup boiling water. Simmer for 20 minutes. Replace the evaporated water, add honey. Some women like to add a little milk, too.

Fruit or Vegetable Juices. These are fine, especially fresh or frozen natural juices, without artificial preservatives and flavorings. If you have access to a juicer, fresh juice is ideal.

Water. Try to have on hand a gallon of spring water or untreated fresh water and drink freely.

Broth. This can be very nourishing, especially during a long labor.

Yogurt or Kefir. These predigested proteins are easily assimilated. During labor, eat yogurt that has been made from whole milk, rather than skim milk or diet yogurt. The high fat content will keep the blood sugar up for a long time. (This is because fats are slower to digest.)

Tigress Smoothie. This is a good source of energy, high in fats and natural sugars. I had a pregnant cat who wouldn't eat anything else for the days before, during, and after giving birth (I didn't put orange juice in hers). (See index for recipe page number).

Papayas. This sweet fruit is high in natural sugars and digestive enzymes for quick and easy assimilation. It has been used by many midwives during labor.

Use of Enemas

If you go into labor and you are constipated, something must be done because a full bowel can cause painful contractions or obstruction.

If you have a regular enema bag, just fill it with a quart of warm water. Otherwise, use a Fleet's disposable phosphate enema, which can be purchased at any drugstore. Don't get the mineral oil enema because this just softens the stool, but doesn't encourage expulsion.

An enema may not be advisable if the waters are broken, because this increases the chance of infection. A last-minute method is to put vaseline up the anus with the finger, which helps to facilitate the passage of stool.

Perineal Massage

As the baby's head is crowning, it is beneficial to take an unopened (and therefore relatively sterile) bottle of vegetable oil such as olive oil, and apply the oil generously while massaging the perineum. The oil can be warmed. Sterile gauze pads can be dipped in the warm oil and placed on the perineum (this could also be done with warm water). This helps loosen up the tissue and makes it more pliable. It helps to prevent tearing and lubricates the passageway, making for a much easier birth. Midwives in the United States, Canada, and Mexico have reported good results with this method.

Perineal massage can also be used before crowning. When the second stage of labor is starting, the midwife can massage the perineum with oil, encouraging the woman to push down toward her fingers.

AFTER THE BIRTH

Baby's First Breath

When your baby emerges from its warm, dark, watery home onto dry land, hopefully into loving hands and gentle, kind vibrations, this new, complete, and aware being does not need to be dangled by its feet like a chicken and given a sharp blow to its bottom to startle it into taking its first gasp.

At this moment, which is so powerful that all astrological and biorhythmic data is based upon it, a healthy baby will usually wrinkle its nose and forehead and breathe without further ado.

But if your little one is not breathing, someone should blow air on its navel and flick the soles of its feet. This will usually stimulate a gasp reflex, which will start the breathing. However, if your baby still does not take a breath, the doctor or midwife may need to clear the airways and give mouth-to-mouth resuscitation.

Cutting the Cord
In some hospitals the umbilical cord is clamped as soon as the baby is born. This deprives the newborn of 20 percent of its blood supply, which is still in the placenta.

An alternate method used by many midwives is to lie the baby across the length of the mother's abdomen (along her waistline), where it will be warm and familiar. Position the baby on its side, with its head down, to assist the drainage of mucus. Cover the baby and the mother with a soft blanket. Then the baby's face may be cleaned and the mucus suctioned from its mouth and nose.

The midwife or doctor can observe and feel the cord. The vein and arteries in the cord lose tone after a few minutes; wait until the cord is done pulsating, then cut and tie it. The end should be rubbed with a disinfectant, such as undiluted apple cider vinegar.

Expelling the Placenta
If the baby nurses, the uterus will contract automatically, which will help to stimulate the delivery of the placenta. Normally, the placenta will come out without any special encouragement within a half hour. If there is a delay beyond this period, the following herbs are helpful.

Angelica (root or seed). If you are using the powder, take four 00 caps, followed by a half cup of hot water. Or sprinkle one teaspoon of powder into one cup of boiling water, and simmer for five minutes. If you are using the whole root or seed, use two teaspoons to a cup of water and simmer for twenty minutes. The placenta usually arrives within five to ten minutes after taking the angelica. One cup of tea should be enough, but you can take more if necessary.

Blue Cohosh. This herb works by contracting the uterus. One cup of tea is usually enough.

> **Blue Cohosh Tea**. Boil 1 cup of water, add 1 teaspoon blue cohosh. Steep in a covered container for 15 minutes. Add 1 teaspoon of peppermint to improve the flavor, if desired.

Some midwives like to carry these herbs in their birth kit in tincture form. Tinctures are easy to administer and fast-acting. Just put a few drops in water or juice and drink, or take the drops directly under the tongue. Tinctures are prepared by adding just enough alcohol to cover the (preferably fresh) herb and letting it sit for about ten days, shaking the bottle each day, and then straining off the alcohol on the last day. Usually five to ten drops are equal to a cup of tea. Tinctures are available in some health food stores. When you buy a tincture, follow the instructions on the bottle since tinctures vary in strength.

Contracting the Uterus

After the birth, the uterus should contract down to a firm ball. The top should be felt at about the level of your navel. If it feels "boggy" or cannot be felt at navel level, deep lower-abdominal massage will help contract the uterus and stop the bleeding. Nursing also causes contractions. As the placenta is delivered, the uterus becomes a bit smaller. It should be about the size and consistency of a grapefruit.

As the milk comes in, replacing the colostrum, the uterus becomes smaller and smaller, until in several weeks it can no longer be felt. If the uterus does not contract adequately, the following teas have been helpful. Drink one cup of blue cohosh tea (recipe above) or birthroot tea.

> **Birthroot Tea**. Boil 1 cup water, add 1 teaspoon of the root, and simmer for 20 minutes.

Nursing After Birth

If your baby wants to suckle, let it take your breast. Then you will be assured of the reality of having given birth and that the child is alive and well. And your child can feel and taste the warmth of its mother and hear her familiar heartbeat.

Based on my own experience at births, and on the use of hypnosis to help people relive their births, in most cases, when a baby is born, it longs for the breast. Like a newborn kitten, it longs for its mother and for her breast. Yet some healthy babies born by natural childbirth do not show an interest in the breast for a half hour or longer. This is not cause for alarm, but the breast should be offered. The sucking reflex is strongest during the first ten minutes after birth.

The symbiotic relationship between mother and child is quite perfect here, where the suckling of the baby directly causes the contraction of the uterus, which assists in the expulsion of the placenta.

One study revealed that infants who were given fifteen to twenty minutes of skin-to-skin and suckling contact with their mother immediately after birth continued to breastfeed for an average of two-and-one-half months longer than the control group of babies who were taken away from their mothers for at least thirty minutes just after birth. Nursing immediately after giving birth enables the mother to establish a good milk supply, because sucking stimulates the release of the pituitary hormone prolactin, which then stimulates secretion of milk.

If your baby does not show an interest in nursing after one day, squeeze your nipple between your thumb and index finger to help it protrude into the baby's mouth, and squeeze your breast to allow a bit of milk to dribble on your baby's lips.

When your baby licks or touches your nipples, prolactin increases in your blood by four to six times the normal concentration. Prolactin is called the love hormone, because it activates close attachment between a mother and her baby.

Eye-to-eye contact between mother and child during breastfeeding can be very rewarding. While you are nursing, the distance between your eyes and your infant's is the exact distance at which newborns can best focus.

When your baby cries, it actually increases the amount of blood flow to your breasts. You might feel your milk coming in, and that will create a pressure which makes you want to nurse.

There are other phenomenon that are harder to explain scientifically. I've known many mothers who experienced a let-down of their milk just as their infant woke up and cried for them—even though the mother was not near the child at the time, and was in fact many miles away.

Bonding

After the birth, many midwives and doctors like to place the infant across the mother's abdomen to keep it warm while they suction the nose and mouth. The mother should see her baby at once to be reassured that it is healthy. Even if it is not healthy, the mother and father need to see and touch their baby. Then they can decide when to hold the child. Sometimes a new mother needs a bit of time to recover from the intensity of the labor before she's ready to embrace her new baby. If her previous child was ill or died, she may be apprehensive about forming this attachment. Let it come in its own time. Hold the child near, but wait until the mother indicates that she is ready to take the baby.

Some mothers experience feeling indifferent when holding their babies—especially those who had their membranes ruptured artificially, or experienced a painful labor, or received a generous dose of Demerol. For many mothers, the affection doesn't develop until some time during the first week—or even later. This may be one reason why many cultures give the mother and baby at least a week alone, so they can have plenty of time to establish the bond which will affect their entire relationship. If the mother forms a deep identification with the baby, this will allow her to meet her infant's needs fairly automatically.

During most of the first hour, newborn babies who have not been drugged tend to remain in a quiet, alert state, with eyes wide open and the ability to respond to their environment. During this time, an infant can see, has visual preferences, and will turn his or her head to the spoken word. This child will actually move in rhythm to his or his mother's voice. After the first hour, infants are in this quiet, alert state only about 10 percent of the time.

It's very rewarding for the parents to see such a responsive baby, so this is the ideal time for bonding. It's a magical time that makes such a powerful impression on parents that they feel a much closer tie to their babies. It's best if mother, father, and baby can be alone together in a separate room during the first hour.

One study showed that when the father was asked to undress his infant twice and to establish eye-to-eye contact with his baby for a total of an hour during the first three days of life, these fathers became much more involved in caring for their infants during the first three months of the babies' lives. And when fathers are given the opportunity to be alone with their newborns, they spend almost the same amount of time as mothers in holding, touching, and looking at these precious new creatures. They are equally sensitive to the baby and just as successful at bottle feeding.

Anthropologist Margaret Mead observed that in societies where men have to leave home to go hunting or do other tasks for long periods, there are taboos against the fathers touching their newborns. Ms. Mead believed that this was done because if new fathers were allowed to fondle their babies they would get so hooked that they would never get out and do their work for society.

According to Dr. Marshall Klaus, the author of *Bonding, The Beginning of Parent-Infant Attachment*, skin-to-skin contact is the best way to make this connection with your newborn. It is extremely satisfying for both the mother and the father to experience holding their nude baby against their nude chests. The human body gives the best form of heat for the newborn; just wrap a receiving blanket or a soft quilt over both of you, and your baby will be perfectly warm.

Klaus emphasizes the importance of eye-to-eye contact, and therefore withholds the application of drops to the baby's eyes until after this initial one-hour time period.

*   *   *

I've pondered on the magical experience of looking into the alert eyes of a healthy newborn baby. These babies often seem like wise and ancient beings. I believe that when we die, the soul lives on, and eventually finds its way into a new body. It is a special privilege to witness this extraordinary combination of innocence and wisdom.

When your baby's eyes meet yours with complete trust, they have an openness which is virtually incomprehensible. In a baby's eyes, we see the miracle of life renewed — an opportunity for a part of ourselves to begin anew, without a backlog of pain and defensiveness.

Seeing our newborn baby is literally falling in love. It is the moment when we perceive that a part of ourself, a part of our very flesh, is at one with Spirit. We see ourselves in our baby's body, and we see a pure spirit in our baby's eyes. We smile at our baby, and Spirit smiles back at us. It is the smile of the one who knows all, who accepts and loves us unconditionally. This pure spirit infuses us with the desire to happily tend to his or her every need, and even to kiss his or her precious little feet.

The mother sees a being who has lived within her body, aware of her every move, a perpetual audience to the drumbeat of her heart, a witness to her every emotion. When this child descends through her birth canal, its adrenalin combines with hers to bring about the contractions that create its birth. And when the child is born, if the child and the mother are fully awake and alert, what a joy it is for these two beings, so beloved to one another, to finally set eyes on one another!

I believe that parents and children choose one another, long before either are born, because of bonds they made in past lives. And so, when you see your baby, there is a part of your subconscious that *recognizes* this being and rejoices to be reunited at last.

But sometimes the past is difficult, and this may explain the ambivalence or even aversion that some parents feel toward their newborns. There is an expectation that all parents will adore their children, yet this isn't always true. If you find that your love doesn't flow toward your child, it may be helpful to explore what your past connection is to this person. A past-life regression may be helpful. In any case, you can be sure that this child will be a teacher for you.

Resting After Childbirth

Many women pride themselves on how quickly they get back on their feet after their baby is born. They point to various native women who literally gave birth in the fields and then went back to work at once. This is considered a great display of strength and good health, and an example to be followed.

Yet I talked to a Chicana woman who returned to work immediately after childbirth, and she said that since she was not able to rest after the birth, and because she tore and was not sewn, she did not heal properly, and intercourse "was not so good" afterwards. She said this was also true of other women she knew.

An astute male nurse observed that the tribes that practiced such behavior were male dominated; the women had to get back to work immediately.

On the other hand, in China, the custom is for a new mother to stay in bed for two weeks before she returns to work. The Hopi Indians kept both the mother and child in bed for a full month after a delivery. The Pomo Indians had birth houses and rest periods after birth. In Czechoslovakia, no woman was allowed to do any work for three weeks after childbirth, and then she was given three months of rest in varying degrees. After the birth, she stayed in a separate birth house, where other women cared for her.

With my first child, I felt very strong. Though I had a difficult, thirty-six-hour labor, I was up and about in two days. I felt fine. Yet I never fully regained the strength I had before my pregnancy. With my last child, I was walking around right after the birth. I rested a lot, but I never stayed in bed. A week after he was born, I took a three hour trip with my baby. There I met a third-generation herbalist from Arkansas. She noticed immediately that my abdomen was still protruding, and she chastised me for being out of bed so early. She was right. Five years later, my abdomen still protruded, and my energy was not what it had been. I think of pregnancy as taking a lot out of me — perhaps it would have been different if I hadn't been so "strong."

Other women have written to me about this:

"I tried to assist too much after one week, even though my husband was around. I had two years of leg pains, low back pains, and a protruding stomach."

*   *   *

"I had a discharge after my baby's birth which lasted about 2½ months (six weeks is normal), partially because I never stayed in bed or rested after my baby's birth (he was born at home), and we moved when he was a month old so I just kept going."

Marj Watkins, herbalist, suggests, "I believe it's best when a new mother has only herself and her baby to care for for the first two weeks. Nurse lying down. Let visitors stay for only fifteen minutes each. Let someone else do the cooking and laundry at least. Don't do any heavy lifting, scrubbing, or mopping until the bleeding ceases. Create a happy calm quiet place for the mother and baby. Gradually resume a full work load over six weeks' time. By then the baby sleeps longer and requires less frequent feedings."

At Fremont Women's Clinic in Seattle, they counsel pregnant women and their partners and friends that after giving birth, a woman should stay in bed or rest as much as she wants. If she feels a strong desire to get up, she should do so, but she should be able to go back to bed as soon as she wants to. It should be arranged so that all tasks can be cheerfully done without any help from the new mother for two full weeks. Then she should be able to slowly resume her daily work, at the pace she chooses for herself.

It's not unreasonable for men to request a pregnancy leave of absence. Men should be able to take two to four weeks off from work, to care for their wife or partner and to get to know their new baby. This is especially important at home births, where the temptation and need to get back into housework is so much greater.

Promoting General Healing

Various women have reported rapid healing of tissues, cessation of bleeding, and ability to resume intercourse in three weeks (instead of the usual four to six weeks) when using the following.

Comfrey, Shepherd's Purse, and Raspberry Leaf Tea. Shepherd's purse is used here to lighten the bleeding, but since blood is the body's natural form of elimination, the shepherd's purse may be omitted after three to seven days, so that some of the bleeding will continue. The comfrey and raspberry may be continued (same proportions) until the discharge stops altogether. Drink up to three cups per day.

> **Comfrey, Shepherd's Purse, and Raspberry Leaf Tea**. Boil 6 cups of water. Add 2 tablespoons comfrey leaves and simmer for 10 minutes. Remove from the heat. Add 2 tablespoons shepherd's purse and 2 tablespoons raspberry leaves. Steep in a covered pot for 5 minutes. Refrigerate what you don't use, and heat as needed.

Cranberry Juice. This is an excellent blood cleanser and purifier of the kidneys and bladder. Some midwives suggest using it after giving birth to cleanse the system. Take three cups per day for three days, then two cups per day for three days, then one cup per day for at least three more days.

Dong Quai. This Chinese herb strengthens the female organs, regulates monthly periods, rebuilds the blood, and helps the mother to regain her strength after the birth of her baby. Nibble on a pea-size piece of the root once or twice a day and let it dissolve slowly in your mouth. Do this for about two weeks after giving birth. Dong Quai is available in many places that sell herbs.

POSSIBLE PROBLEMS

Premature Labor

If you go into labor more than two weeks before your due date, especially if you seem to be carrying a small baby, this could result in having a premature baby. If the contractions continue, consult your doctor or midwife. In order to stop the contractions, you could drink up to three glasses of wine in the course of the day. This is not ordinarily advisable during pregnancy, but it's less drastic than the medication that is often given to women who go into premature labor.

How to Bring On Labor

Don't tamper with due dates unnecessarily. The fruit ripens in its own time; the day and time of birth have potent astrologic and biorhythmic implications. But sometimes a trusted midwife or doctor may feel that nature needs a little help. Then we are blessed with gentle herbs to help us in this process.

The body and mind work together, and before intervening, it's a good idea to try and find out if there are emotional factors that could be slowing down the birthing process. Sit down with yourself (or with a close friend or your partner or midwife—someone you feel you can share your deepest secrets with), and explore every possible fear or misgiving you may have about giving birth. Dredge up the irrational, the silly, and the embarrassing. If you're afraid, tell yourself: "I will neither fear nor desire any of these thoughts. I will just let them pass through." You might want to write down all your thoughts as they occur to you. When you're quite sure that you've dredged up all of them, look deep inside and you may find another one squirming around in there. Then look at everything you've brought up, openly and honestly. You may have found some things you need to change. You could make some realistic promises to yourself concerning the future. Usually, fear thrives on darkness, and once it's brought into the light, it loses its power. Fear can easily hold back your labor.

You may also want to tune in to your baby and discuss your misgivings with her or him. You may want to prepare this new and ancient being for the life ahead of you both. Some women maintain this kind of rapport throughout their pregnancy. Don't be overly concerned about whether you're really communicating or not. Just give your fantasy free reign, and go where it takes you.

If intervention still seems necessary, you can try the following.

Birthroot (Bethroot, Trillium). Birthroot is an endangered herb. It takes seven years to produce its one and only flower. If you gather your own, take just one whole plant. Try to find one that grows among others, rather than in isolation. There is some disagreement about whether the purple or the white flower is the strongest. John Lust writes about the hormonal properties of the purple trillium, but Indians preferred the white flower for women's ailments.

Birthroot Tea. Boil 1 cup water and add 2 teaspoons fresh, chopped root or 1 teaspoon dried root. Simmer for 20 minutes. Drink one to two cups per day.

Placenta Previa

If the baby is being delivered at home, and the placenta comes before the baby, this is a severe emergency and the mother must be taken to the hospital immediately. It is possible to stop the labor altogether by having the mother

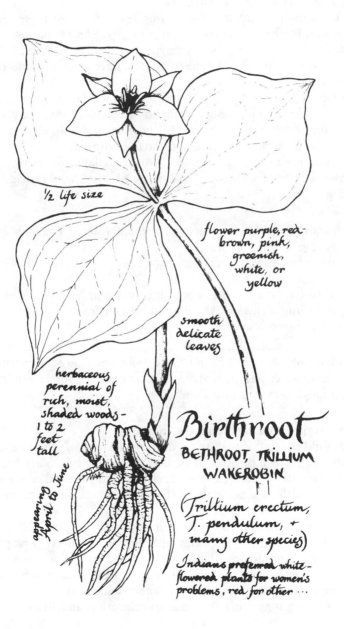

½ life size

flower purple, red-
brown, pink,
greenish,
white, or
yellow

smooth
delicate
leaves

herbaceous
perennial of
rich, moist,
shaded woods -
1 to 2
feet
tall

appearing
April to June

Birthroot
BETHROOT, TRILLIUM
WAKEROBIN

(Trillium erectum,
T. pendulum, +
many other species)

Indians preferred white-
flowered plants for women's
problems, red for other ...

drink as much as a half bottle of brandy or whiskey. This should *never* be done under ordinary circumstances, since it is taxing to the baby's immature liver. However, in this situation, it may be a life-saving measure.

Speeding Up a Slow Labor

Begin by spending time talking about your fears. Some of these fears may seem irrelevant, but be sure to take them seriously. Some common fears are, "How will my family feel about my having a home birth?" and "How will my man respond to the baby?" Once these fears are expressed and released, labor often resumes dramatically.

Another subtle cause of a slow labor occurs when a woman has chosen a home birth in order to please her husband or friends, but she really doesn't feel secure about delivering at home. In these cases, labor will resume dramatically as soon as the woman arrives at the hospital.

Relaxation is an important element in helping labor on its way. A long warm shower can be very relaxing, and many hospitals now provide this for the laboring woman.

Blue Cohosh Tea. This is effective for some women. You may drink one or two cups, one cup per hour.

If vomiting occurs after drinking the tea, don't panic; vomiting is normal during transition.

Herbalist Mrs. Grieve writes about blue cohosh: "In use it is preferable to Ergot, expediting delivery, where delay results from debility, fatigue or want of uterine nervous energy."

Blue Cohosh Tea. Cover 1½ teaspoons of blue cohosh with 1 cup boiling water and let it steep in a covered pot for 15 minutes. Use as much honey as you like.

Promoting Relaxation or Sleep

Sometimes mild contractions drag on and on. I know of many cases where labor continued for two or three days, and the waters still didn't break. The midwife and/or doctor kept close supervision, and the mother stayed calm and was able to deliver a perfectly normal baby in the surroundings of her choice.

Keeping the blood sugar up with kefir or yogurt, keeping well-nourished with hearty broths, and keeping calm with herbal teas are very helpful. But sometimes a long and difficult labor will respond best to a nap. A woman in labor who is under great tension can awaken from a nap refreshed and in much higher spirits, with more forceful contractions.

The following suggestions are aids to relaxation and sleep.

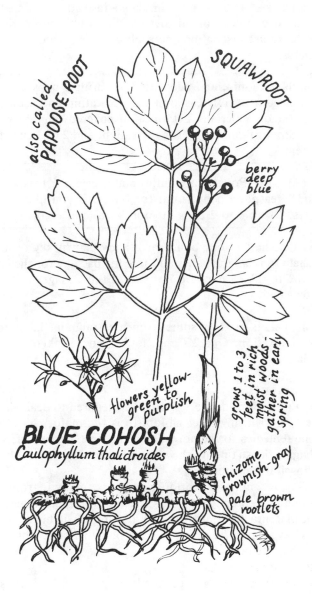

also called
PAPOOSE ROOT

SQUAWROOT

berry
deep
blue

flowers yellow-
green to
purplish

grows 1 to 3
feet in rich
moist woods -
gather in early
spring

BLUE COHOSH
Caulophyllum thalictroides

rhizome
brownish-gray

pale brown
rootlets

Valerian, Catnip, and Scullcap Tea. Valerian is an excellent muscle relaxant, but some people have a bad reaction to it, and get a stomachache, dizziness, or nausea. Others are stimulated instead of calmed. If you're repulsed by the strong odor of this herb and if you've never tried it before, it may be better to use just catnip and scullcap, one teaspoon each and brew for five minutes.

Valerian, Catnip, and Scullcap Tea. Bring 2 cups of water to a boil, and pour over 1 teaspoon each of catnip and scullcap and ½ teaspoon of Valerian. Let brew in covered container for 20 minutes. Strain. Drink 1 cup for relaxation, and 2 to 3 cups to promote sleep.

Catnip Tea. Pour 1 cup boiling water over 1½ teaspoons catnip. Add 1 teaspoon peppermint for flavor, if you like. Steep for 5 minutes. Drink 1 to 2 cups or more as a mild relaxant.

Brandy. One-half to one ounce of brandy or whiskey or a small glass of wine can help to relax the pelvis and free the passage for the baby. It may also enable you to take a nap. Do not exceed this dosage, or the baby may be born intoxicated.

Calcium. This is used by some women throughout labor to ease pain and promote relaxation. One 250 mg. tablet can be taken every half hour throughout labor.

Hemorrhaging

Anyone planning a home delivery should be prepared to deal with this emergency, since hemorrhaging after childbirth is the major cause of maternal deaths. Home remedies for hemorrhaging can be extremely effective, but if the hemorrhaging doesn't diminish within five minutes, the mother should be taken to a hospital immediately.

Marion Toepke, nurse-practitioner and nurse-midwife from the Frontier Nursing Service in Kentucky, suggests the following techniques.

1. If the placenta has been delivered, the uterus will be the size of a small cantaloupe. Grasp it *tightly*, with one hand on either side. This pressure will help to stop the bleeding.

2. Note the time.

3. Have someone else try to get the baby to nurse. This causes contractions, which help ease the bleeding.

4. Give shepherd's purse tea (see below).

5. After five minutes, release the pressure on the uterus.

By this time, the bleeding should have stopped, or eased significantly. If not, prepare to go to a hospital at once. Meanwhile, massage the uterus

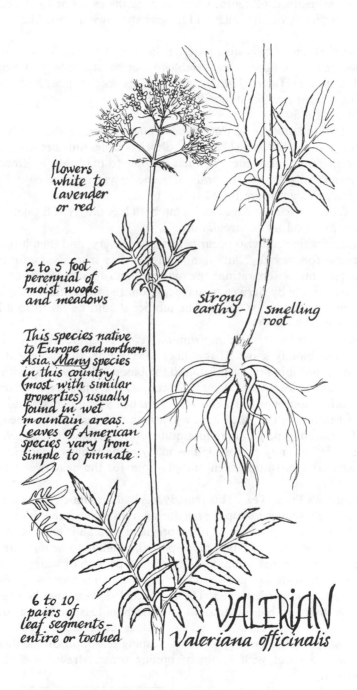

flowers
white to
lavender
or red

2 to 5 foot
perennial of
moist woods
and meadows

strong
earthy-   smelling
root

This species native
to Europe and northern
Asia. Many species
in this country
(most with similar
properties) usually
found in wet
mountain areas.
Leaves of American
species vary from
simple to pinnate:

6 to 10
pairs of
leaf segments-
entire or toothed

VALERIAN
Valeriana officinalis

by kneading it firmly. This helps to close down the blood vessels and to expel pieces of the retained placenta, which may be the cause of the bleeding. Or have the mother sit on the toilet and massage her own uterus. She should not be left alone.

If hemorrhaging continues, there is danger of shock. This occurs when the blood vessels collapse. It's advisable to monitor the pulse and blood pressure. If the pulse is faster than normal, or if the mother goes into shock, the following actions are recommended.

1. Give fluids.

2. Have the mother lie flat; remove pillows from under her head. Elevate her legs to get blood to her brain. Shock is dangerous because the blood vessels close down, and since the blood supply to the brain is already minimal, this can easily deprive the brain of needed oxygen and glucose. Elevating the legs helps to get more blood to the brain.

3. Take two ace bandages and wrap both legs snugly. This helps to keep two pints of blood up in circulation.

Hemorrhaging can also occur *before* the delivery, and then it is extremely dangerous for the baby. Any significant bleeding from the uterus indicates that the placenta is separating: the maternal and fetal surfaces are coming apart. Since the baby derives its oxygen from the placenta, this may result in possible retardation or death. The mother should be taken to a hospital immediately.

On the other hand, bleeding from the cervix is natural during labor, and it's known as bloody show. If the labor is very fast, the bloody show may be excessive, but it is not harmful, and the blood will be mixed with mucus.

How much bleeding is normal? Of course, this will vary from one woman to another, and it will depend on how much you move around. For example, when you lie flat, the blood will accumulate but may not be expelled. Then if you stand up, you may lose quite a bit of blood. But general guidelines are that you may go through as many as six sanitary pads in the first four hours after birth and then one per hour for the next twelve hours.

Shepherd's Purse Tea. This remedy has had dramatic results for numerous women. You can make up the tea during transition, so that it's ready after the birth. If it's a long labor, or if the pregnant woman is anemic, or if there are any other factors that might predispose the woman to hemorrhaging, you can make a stronger tea—about two teaspoons per cup of water. One cup of tea is usually enough, but use up to four cups per day if necessary. *Note:* This herb is a common garden weed. The leaves and flowers may be used. If it's used fresh, then double the amount (two heaping teaspoons per cup).

Shepherd's Purse Tea. Use 1 heaping teaspoon of shepherd's purse and cover with 1 cup of boiling water. Brew for 5 to 30 minutes.

Cayenne. When hemorrhaging occurs, immediately give ½ teaspoon of cayenne. Repeat this every half hour for up to three hours if necessary. Cayenne can be given in 00 gelatin capsules (each capsule holds ¼ teaspoon), or it can be taken (¼ teaspoon at a time) by placing the cayenne at the end of a butter knife and dropping it on the back of the tongue, where there aren't many taste buds. Then swallow it down with water. Cayenne is available in grocery stores and health food stores.

Minor Tears

Minor tears are nicks in the perineum, up to one-half inch, that do not require stitches. Large openings should be stitched within eight hours of the delivery. One midwife writes: "The mother of the third baby I delivered had a tear just longer than one-quarter inch and we left it, but it healed with a little flap, which she feels, and finds irritating. (It also kept opening initially, and took quite a while to heal.)"

To promote rapid healing of minor tears, the following remedies have proven effective.

Comfrey. This herb promotes fast healing, and is good for the minor tears of childbirth. Comfrey ointment may be applied. Some women like to use a piece of the fresh green leaf, crushed to release the juices, and placed directly over the tear and under the pad. Or a tea can be made with comfrey leaf.

> **Comfrey Tea**. Simmer 1 tablespoon dried or 2 tablespoon fresh comfrey leaves in 1 cup of water for 10 minutes. If comfrey root is used, use 1 tablespoon dried or 2 tablespoon fresh root and simmer in 1¼ cups of water for 20 minutes. A soft cloth can be dipped into the warm strained tea and applied to the tears. This may be done three or more times per day.

Light. Exposure to the sun, or to a sunlamp, or close exposure (about one foot) to a forty-watt light bulb has helped to promote healing. This can be done for about ten minutes, three times a day. If you are using a sunlamp, expose the tear at about three feet, three to five minutes, two or three times a day.

Stitches

Any tears that are one-quarter inch or longer should be sutured within eight hours after giving birth. When stitches are necessary, there will be some additional discomfort on the following days, because the stitches tend to itch or hurt. A ginger compress helps to relieve the discomfort.

Ginger Compress. To make the compress, take two tablespoons freshly grated ginger or one tablespoon dried ginger pieces or two teaspoons ginger powder. Simmer in one cup water for twenty minutes. Strain. Dip a clean washcloth in the hot tea (not too hot) and apply to the navel, working slowly down to and over the stitches. Dip and wring the cloth again whenever it cools.

Pain on Urination

Since urine is acidic, it often causes burning pain to the perineum if there has been any tearing or stitches.

Drink a lot of fluids after giving birth to dilute the urine and make urination less painful.

An enterprising doctor suggests this ingenious device: Cut out one of the egg holders from a plastic or cardboard egg carton. Cut a hole at the bottom. Insert the smaller end between the labia and around the urethra and try to urinate through the hole. This should keep the urine from getting on the tear. He suggests trying this before the baby is born, so you can get the hang of it.

Excessive Discharge

If the bleeding stays red and does not turn pink and diminish after three days, and if the uterus remains tender or painful, this could be a sign that there are still pieces of placenta in the uterus. Angelica has been given by many midwives with excellent results.

Angelica (root or seed). If you're using the powder, take four 00 caps, followed by ½ cup warm water. Or make a tea.

Repeat the dosage two or three times per day until the discharge stops. Angelica encourages the movement of pieces of placenta out of the uterus, perhaps by contractions, as with the retained placenta.

Be sure to get plenty of rest, elevate your feet, and call your doctor or midwife, since this condition could lead to a serious infection.

> **Angelica Tea**. Sprinkle 1 teaspoon of powder into 1 cup of boiling water and simmer for 5 minutes. If you are using the whole root or seed, use 2 teaspoons to 1 cup water and simmer for 20 minutes.

Postpartum Blues

This phenomenon is seen less frequently after home births, or births that are attended by a midwife or labor coach, and births where drugs are not used. Klaus says, "We do not know the causes of postpartum blues, but our observations lead us to speculate that mother-infant separation, the assignment of most of the care-giving responsibilities to 'experts,' the concerns about ability to care for the newborn at home, and the limiting of visitors are major factors."

IF THE BABY DIES

When I was pregnant with my second child, we were living in New Mexico. We moved to a house that was five minutes from the local hospital. We had a small farm in the desert, and my husband had to irrigate every day, carrying heavy barrels of water.

One day he had to work late and was unable to return home on time to irrigate. I was strong and believed I could do anything—even though I was eight months pregnant. So I carried the heavy barrels of water.

We found a midwife to deliver the baby at home. When the due date came and passed, I wasn't concerned because I knew several women who delivered two to four weeks late. After two weeks, the doctor at the hospital wanted to induce labor, but I refused.

Two weeks later I entered my tenth month and I went into labor. I was overjoyed to be at home. The midwife was wonderful. My husband was supportive. My son was there. I was relaxed and confident.

I labored for eighteen hours, and it seemed short compared to the thirty-six hours of my first birth. Finally the midwife said I could push. I could feel the baby bursting through, and I gave an incredible yell, and delivered my baby.

I was flat on my back (in 1970 we weren't conscious about other positions). I couldn't see what was going on. I heard a strange noise, like someone trying to blow up a balloon. Time passed. I just lay there, in a kind of stupor.

Then a voice said, "Your baby was born dead."

Born—dead. I could barely comprehend what it meant. Her body was whisked away. I never saw her.

They meant well. They wanted to spare me the pain.

But how can you mourn for what you haven't seen? For the feeling of life in your belly that is now nothingness? For the anticipation of dreams that are now a charade?

The midwife cleaned me up hastily. She was shocked, and afraid of being charged with manslaughter. My husband drove me to the hospital. They were angry with us. The doctor gave me antibiotics. No one was kind to me. They examined the baby and said she'd been dead for at least three days. The cord was wrapped round her neck seven times.

We went home empty-handed. They wouldn't even let us bury her on our own land.

I felt crazy for about a year. Whenever I saw a baby, I would touch it and fondle it and talk about my little girl. My only comfort was that I had had a home birth. That had been a beautiful experience. If it had happened in the hospital, it would have been unbearable.

It was excruciating to have carried life in my belly and then given birth to a lifeless child. My body was prepared to nurse and mother a newborn child. My breasts were full of milk for that child. My whole being was ready to hold my baby and bring this new person into my life. It was exceedingly painful to find myself empty-armed, with nothing at all to show for so many months of waiting and preparing.

And it was no easy thing to explain to well-meaning relatives and friends who called on the phone or stopped me on the street to inquire if the baby had come yet.

Many years later I read an interview with Elisabeth Kübler-Ross, the psychiatrist who pioneered a new consciousness about working with the dying. She spoke about working with parents who have experienced the death of a small child. She suggested that the funeral director should allow the parents to prepare their child for the casket. She suggested that the parents bathe the child and put on its pajamas and brush its hair, as if they were putting the child to sleep.

"My God," I thought, "If my husband and I had done that, we'd have cried and cried and cried!"

Then I realized that was exactly what we avoided doing. That was why our grief went on and on and on.

Kübler-Ross said it was normal to feel shocked and numb when someone dies. It was normal to feel pain and anger, and it was important to express those feelings. She urged medical people to avoid prescribing sedatives which prevent people from feeling these feelings. She described cultures where people wailed at funerals and she suggested that hospitals should have screaming rooms.

I went to two of her workshops, and then to a psychodrama workshop. I wrote the script for my own psychodrama, and other people played the roles of the people who were present when my baby was born dead. I played myself.

This time when they took the baby away, I insisted that they bring her back. "I want to see my baby!" I demanded. They brought her to me. It was a doll, all wrapped up in a receiving blanket.

They handed her to me, and I uncovered her face. The doll looked distorted. That didn't matter to me. This was my baby. I touched her little face. I cried. I hugged her. I held her and rocked her and cried and cried.

Finally, after a long time, I was able to let her go. But I've never forgotten that baby.

It was a great help to re-live that experience. To give myself permission to cry. To take my power to hold my own child. To face her death. I'm grateful for that opportunity.

After that, my life became richer. I stopped holding onto old grief and allowing it to permeate the present. I had more energy for my other children (by this time I had another son).

*   *   *

Since then I've had the opportunity to help many parents to work through the death of their babies, and I've worked with many midwives who have done the same.

If your baby dies, the attitude of your care-givers will have a profound effect on you. Doctors and nurses who express sadness or empathy will be appreciated. Unfortunately, doctors may feel guilty about the baby's death, which puts them in a poor position to be comforting.

If the baby was delivered by a midwife at home, then she or he is in possible jeopardy, but most midwives will see a family through every step of their grieving. Yet I know too many midwives who ended their career after experiencing the delivery of a dead baby. Care-givers should bear in mind that they, too, need time to grieve. They need to grieve the loss of their image as one who brings forth life, and to deal with the disappointment, anger, guilt, and shock of delivering a stillborn.

There are two ways that parents and professionals can deal with death: One is to become numb to it—cold and uninvolved, so that it does not touch them. It is the way of denial, and those who take this route will bring that same lack of emotion into their private lives.

The other way is, as Kübler-Ross suggests, to "drain the pool of sorrow." Most of us have unfinished business, old grief that we have not fully released. One death reminds us of another death, or loss. When we truly finish the process of grieving all the old losses, and cry out the tears and scream the screams, then we are ready to be fully present.

Many nurses and midwives now understand that you will probably want to bond with your dead baby, even though it is terribly painful. The pain enables you to feel your feelings and pass through the stages of grieving. Otherwise there is emptiness without evidence of anything to grieve for, and the grieving often becomes pathological and the mother, especially, suffers mentally.

It is becoming increasingly common for midwives or nurses to offer to photograph the baby who has died. Some will also take plaster-of-paris footprints as a keepsake of the baby. A trip to the mortuary is not uncommon, where the midwife goes with the mother or parents, and they are allowed to undress and touch their infant. This is difficult after an autopsy, but even then it is better than not doing it at all. Whenever possible, it's best if the parents can handle the baby before the autopsy.

When there is fear of how the baby will look, it's good for the midwife (or friend, or nurse) to look first, and then the parents might want to ask questions and be prepared before they feel ready to look. If there are parts of the baby that are especially difficult to look at, the assistant can cover these parts with the receiving blanket before offering the baby to the parents.

Many people consider this bizarre. "Why add to your suffering?" they ask. But it doesn't add to the suffering—it makes the suffering tangible, and this helps us to express our feelings, and when the feelings are expressed, they pass, and then we can move on with our lives.

It's good if close relatives and friends can see the baby. This helps them to share in the grief, and to be a greater comfort to the parents. Otherwise it's difficult, when they've never known this baby for whom the parents grieve.

Another ritual that helps to make the death more real is a funeral. The most rewarding funerals occur in communities where people know the parents and care about them, and each person is encouraged to speak from the heart and say or bring something personal to share in the ritual. It is satisfying when the coffin (if there is a coffin) can actually be lowered into the ground, and each person who feels close to the baby or to the parents can take a spadeful of dirt and toss it on the grave.

You may want the grave site to be fairly accessible because visits to your baby's grave can be comforting.

You need to know that your friends care about you. You need permission to talk about your baby, about your lost hopes and dreams. And friends can help by making it clear that they're willing to listen and to acknowledge the pain.

In a sense, you are grieving for the loss of a part of yourself (flesh of your flesh), as well as the image of yourself as a parent, and the myriad of lost dreams. And the mother is grieving over the failure of her body to work as it was meant to.

I urge well-meaning friends and care-givers to refrain from telling these parents that "It's probably for the best," or "Every cloud has a silver lining," or "You'll get over it soon," or "You can always have another baby." The work at hand is to mourn the baby who has died, and it is often seen as an insult to the memory of this irreplaceable being to suggest that it can be easily replaced.

However, many women do get pregnant soon after their baby has died. They hope to find comfort in the new child, but this is not advisable, because grieving requires energy, and a pregnant woman needs to give her energy to her new baby. I urge couples to wait at least six months, or until they feel that they have reached a point of acceptance about their baby's death before attempting a new pregnancy.

Men in our culture have a hard time expressing their feelings — especially by crying. But grief that is held in makes you hard and rigid and eventually it makes you mean. And women desperately need to share their grief with their men. I urge fathers to allow themselves to feel their grief, their tears, their loss. You do *not* need to be a pillar of strength for your family.

In fact, if you keep a stiff upper lip, and if you have boy-children, you will be unconsciously telling your children that this is the proper way for a man to grieve. Your behavior will be a model for them on how to deal with death in the future. If you dare to express your feelings, you will be giving them permission to do so also. Children *need* to see you fall apart, and then pick up the pieces. They need to see that you can feel your feelings and still survive.

Talk to your children about what has happened. Express your feelings. If at all possible, don't send them away to stay with friends or relatives. If you send them away, they'll feel like they're being punished. They'll feel guilty—as if somehow they were responsible for the baby's death—and the natural jealousy that children feel toward their potential siblings adds to such a fantasy.

Include your children in the funeral—a ritual of some kind is important to children. It helps them to acknowledge and express their own feelings, and it's a way of honoring life. That's important to them. If possible, have a close friend of the family present at the funeral to be with the children and to answer questions—you may be too lost in your grief to want to do that.

Try to take time off work. Give yourself time to mope around the house. Don't choose this time to take on new projects or a new job, which happens all too often when men (and women) are unable to face their emotions. Talk about it. Talk and talk and talk. You might think that will make it worse, but actually, it makes the pain go away faster.

I have been emphasizing the stillborn child, but most of the same suggestions apply to an early infant death or even a miscarriage.

If it is inevitable that the child is going to die soon, and if the little one is connected to tubes and needles, many parents have found that it is rewarding to take the baby off of the life support system and hold this child in their arms so that he or she can feel the comfort of their love, and they can share their love with this precious being, even if only for a few hours.

A wonderful book, which has been of great help to parents who are grieving, is *Ended Beginnings, Healing Childbearing Losses*, by Claudia Panuthos and Catherine Romeo.

REFERENCES

Nancy Wainer Cohen and Lois J. Estner, *Silent Knife* (Bergin & Garvey Publishers, 1983).

Adelle Davis, *Let's Get Well* (Harcourt, Brace and World, 1965).

M. Grieve, *A Modern Herbal* (Dover Publications, 1971).

International Childbirth Education Association, "Update on Breastfeeding," *ICEA Review*, (Spring) 1978.

Marshall H. Klaus, M.D. and John H. Kennell, M.D., *Bonding, The Beginnings of Parent-Infant Attachment* (C.V. Mosby Co., 1983).

John Lust, N.D., *The Herb Book* (Bantam Books, 1974).

"Rigid Hospital Routine May Hinder Breast-Feeding," *Sexual Medicine Today*, November 1978.

Time Magazine, 113, No. 6, February 5, 1979.

Thomas Verny, M.D. with John Kelly, *The Secret Life of the Unborn Child* (Collins Publishers, 1981).

Conclusion

It's spring now and from my window I can still see snow on the mountain across the lake. Already the chives are a foot high in the herb garden. I keep the herbs near the kitchen door, so I can have culinary herbs and peppermint in easy reach.

But most of the medicinal herbs I gather in the nearby woods, or in areas within a few hours of here. Wherever I live, I try to learn about the local herbs, often substituting them for store-bought ones. There are only a few that I depend upon which don't grow locally.

In the spring, I gather elder flowers. In the summer I get red clover, shepherd's purse, mullein, wild ginger, and yarrow. That's when I make my salves with comfrey leaves and plantain.

In the late summer, I gather chicory, elder berries, mullein flowers, and hops.

In the fall, I gather the roots: comfrey, dandelion, echinacea, blackberry, and Oregon grape root. Oregon grape root makes a good substitute for goldenseal. I peel off the yellow bark of the root, which contains hydrastine — one of the primary active ingredients in goldenseal. This year I'll be in visiting in northeastern California where I'll gather ephedra.

Best of all are the wonderful excursions up the mountain where the juniper berries and uva-ursi grow. You can see the whole valley from there, and it's a wonderful place to watch the sunset.

As a day comes to an end, and as a year comes to an end, so too this book must end. Over the years, so many midwives, herbalists, and other people have shared their knowledge with me. I'm grateful that they entrusted me with this gift, and I hope I've done justice to it.

To Your Health,

Joy Gardner

PREGNANCY

The Pregnancy After 30 Workbook, A Program for Safe Childbearing No Matter What Your Age, Gail Sforza Brewer (Rodale Press, 1978). Takes the emphasis off of age and puts it onto general health, diet, exercise, and avoidance of drugs. Describes the work that Gail and Tom Brewer have done with women over thirty and gives encouraging statistics. The same guidelines can be used for teenage mothers.

What Every Pregnant Woman Should Know: The Truth About Diets and Drugs in Pregnancy, Gail Sforza Brewer, with Tom Brewer (Penguin, 1985). The importance of good nutrition during pregnancy with an emphasis on preventing toxemia through nutrition.

As You Eat, So Your Baby Grows, Nikki Goldbeck (Ceres Press, 1980). A concise pamphlet that provides a good guide to nutrition during pregnancy.

Essential Exercises for the Childbearing Year, 2nd edition, by Elizabeth Noble (Houghton Mifflin, 1982). A guide to understanding and coping with the changes of pregnancy.

Transformation Through Birth, A Woman's Guide, Claudia Panuthos (Bergin and Garvey, 1984). An excellent wholistic guide for childbirth, complete with chapters on preparation for birth through the use of visualization and release.

Pregnancy as Healing, Vol. I., Gayle Peterson and Lewis Mehl (Mindbody, 1984). Unites emotional and spiritual aspects with the intimately physical experience of childbearing.

You're Not Too Old to Have a Baby, Jane Price (Penguin, 1978). Good information on delaying parenthood until after age thirty.

The Secret Life of the Unborn Child, Thomas Verny, M.D., with John Kelly (Dell, 1986). Gives firm evidence of how the mother's emotional and physical well-being or lack of it influences the emotional and physical outcome of the newborn—and of the adult that child becomes.

Nourishing Your Unborn Child, Phyllis Williams (Avon, 1982). A complete guide to nutrition during pregnancy and after childbirth, with menus and recipes.

BIRTH

Active Birth, Janet and Arthur Balaskas (McGraw-Hill, 1983). Giving birth on your own two feet with the complete freedom to use your body the way you want. This book will give you supportive tools to achieve what you want for yourself.

Birth Trap, Yvonne Brackbill, June Rice, and Diony Young (Warner, 1984). An exposé of current obstetrical high-tech birthing practices. Well-researched and very perceptive.

Silent Knife: Cesarean Prevention and Vaginal Birth After Cesarean, Nancy Wainer Cohen and Lois J. Estner (Bergin & Garvey, 1983). Comprehensive up-to-date information about all aspects of cesarean birth and prevention. A long book, but highly readable, supportive, and cuttingly humorous.

The Rights of the Pregnant Parent, Valmai Howe Elkins (Shocken, 1985). Prepared childbirth and how to communicate with medical professionals. Emphasizes how to have a supportive doctor, with family-centered care, and the kind of childbirth you want.

Spiritual Midwifery, Ina May Gaskin (Book Publishing Co., rev. 1980). Inspiring accounts of home birthing at The Farm, a religious community in Tennessee that is non-interventionist and has extraordinary birth statistics.

The Complete Book of Pregnancy and Childbirth, Sheila Kitzinger (Knopf, 1980). Comprehensive guide to pregnancy and childbirth.

Prenatal Yoga and Natural Birth, Jeannine Parvatti (North Atlantic, 1986). Yoga exercises that are safe for pregnant women. Lots of photographs.

Childbirth With Insight, Elizabeth Noble (Houghton Mifflin, 1983). Encourages expectant parents to develop the self-reliance and personal responsibility to plan their own birth experience.

Birth Reborn, Michel Odent (Pantheon Books, 1984). French physician Odent describes his inspiring clinic in Pithiviers, France, where women are encouraged to labor as they wish. Different labor positions and delivery methods are described.

Birthing Normally: A Personal Growth Approach to Childbirth, 2nd edition, Gayle H. Peterson (Mindbody Press, 1984). A wholistic approach to prenatal care which gives the process of birthing back to the woman who gives birth.

Cesarean Birth: Risk and Culture, Gayle Peterson and Lewis Mehl (1985). Information on cesarean birth, interventions, family roles, and more. Based on the philosophy of uniting emotional and spiritual aspects of life and childbearing.

BREASTFEEDING

The Experience of Breastfeeding, Sheila Kitzinger (Penguin Books, 1982). A simple book with lots of good basic information on breastfeeding and related topics.

The Womanly Art of Breastfeeding, 3rd edition, La Leche League International (New American Library, 1981). The classic bible of breastfeeding. A pleasure to read.

MISCELLANEOUS

Premature Babies, A Handbook for Parents, Sherri Nance (Priam Books, 1982). Plenty of information and support in a format that is easy to read and understand.

A Child is Born, Lennart Nilsson (Dell, 1977). The best possible way to comprehend exactly what is going on inside your body as your baby develops from month to month.

Having Twins: A Parent's Guide to Pregnancy, Birth, and Early Parenthood, Elizabeth Noble (Houghton Mifflin, 1980). Prenatal care, parenting tips, and fascinating facts dealing with multiple births.

Ended Beginnings—Healing Childbearing Losses, Claudia Panuthos and Catherine Romeo (Bergin and Garvey, 1984). Speaks to parents who are grieving the loss of a child—through miscarriage, stillbirth, sudden infant death, abortion, or the choice of adoption.

Appendix II
Identification and Safety/Toxicity
Status Of Herbs Listed in this Book

The following table was prepared with the help of Dr. Doel D. Soerjarto, Ph.D. in plant toxonomy at Harvard University. The common names of plants and their probable scientific name are both given. The scientific names are italicized, and the letters that follow the names refer to the botantists who named the plant; this is done to avoid confusion.

For regulatory purposes, the U.S. Food and Drug Administration uses the GRAS (Generally Recognized as Safe) proviso of the Food, Drug and Cosmetic Act; that is, any plant that was recognized as GRAS in 1958 is okay to sell and use (within specific restrictions of doses or concentration stated in the act) if listed as GRAS.

Common Name	Scientific Name	Comments
Aloe	*Aloe Vera* (L.) Burm. f.	External use is okay.
Angelica	*Angelica archangelica* L.	Has GRAS status.
Birthroot	*Trillium erectum* L.	Not GRAS, but no reason to suspect toxicity.
Black haw	*Viburnum prunifolium* L.	GRAS.
Blessed thistle	*Cnicus benedictus* L.	GRAS.
Blue cohosh	*Caulophyllum thalictroides* (L.)	Not GRAS. Could be unsafe, but depends on the dose.
Catnip	*Nepeta cataria* L.	Not GRAS, but no evidence of toxicity in animals or humans.
Cayenne	*Capsicum frutescens* L.	GRAS.

189

Comfrey	*Symphytum officinale* L.	Not GRAS. Extracts cause cancer in lab animals fed orally. Active compounds are known. Presence of active compounds is variable, probably depending on where plant is grown. Roots are loaded with the active compounds; leaves only traces to none. External use is okay.
Desert sagebrush	*Artemesia tridenta*	
Dong quai	Probably *Angelica polymorpha* Maxim. var. *sinensis* (Oliver [= *Anglica sinensis*] Diels)	Not GRAS. Probably safe.
Flaxseed	*Linum usitatissimum* L.	Not GRAS, but seeds used commonly as a laxative; could be irritating.
Garlic	*Allium sativum* L.	GRAS. Recommended to be placed in the vagina. Very careful to give precautions against irritant effect.
Ginger	*Zingiber offinale* Roscoe	GRAS.
Marijuana	*Cannabis sativa* L.	Illegal. Not GRAS. Not advisable for pregnant women.
Peppermint	*Mentha X piperita* L.	GRAS.
Pulsatilla	*Pulsatilla nigricans* Storcke	Not GRAS. A homeopathic remedy and thus should have no toxicity.

Raspberry leaf	*Rubus ideaus* L.	Not GRAS, but no animal or human toxicities reported.
Sage	*Salvia officinalis* L.	
Scullcap	*Scutellaria lateriflora* L.	Not GRAS, but no animal or human toxicities reported.
Shepherd's purse	*Capsella bursa* pastoris (L.) Medic	Not GRAS, but no animal or human toxicities reported.
Slippery elm	*Ulmus rubra* Mohl. (= *Ulmus fulva* Michx.)	Not GRAS, but safe for use as recommended.
Squaw vine	*Mitchella repens* L.	Not GRAS, but no animal or human toxicities reported.
Spikenard	*Aralia racemosa* L.	Not GRAS, but probably safe.
Star of Bethlehem	*Orinthogalum umbellatum* L.	Not GRAS. Used as Bach remedy; too dilute to be toxic.
Valerian	*Valeriana officinalis* L.	GRAS

Appendix III
About Homeopathy

This is a branch of medicine that is not widely recognized by the medical profession, despite the fact that all homeopaths are doctors and homeopathy is simply their field of specialization. Homeopathy uses homeopathic preparations, which are derived from plant, mineral, or animal sources. These preparations are chosen according to the principle of "Let like be treated by likes." For example, epilepsy (a convulsive disease) may be treated by a plant which, in large doses, would produce convulsions. A very minute amount of this plant would be combined with a much larger amount of inert material (such as alcohol), and this would then be triturated or rubbed down by a machine so that the two substances were finely mixed. This produces a potentized remedy that has a more powerful curative reaction in the body than a equivalent quantity of the original crude substance, and yet it is harmless. For example, homeopathic (or potentized) poison ivy is sometimes used to treat allergy to poison ivy.

Potencies are designated by a numeral and the letter X and follow the decimal scale. Therefore, 1X indicates 1/10 or 1 part active substance to 10 parts inert substance; 2X indicates 1/100 or 1 part active substance to 100 parts inert substance; 3X indicates 1/1000 or 1 part active per 1,000 parts inactive. Each substance is triturated for eight hours for each successive reduction, which results in an infinitesimal breakdown of active ingredients, permitting ready assimilation into the cells of the body.

Appendix IV
Aluminum

When preparing tea (or anything else), always avoid aluminum. According to Dr. H. Tomlinson, author of *Aluminum Utensils and Disease*, one out of two people he tested were aluminum-sensitive. While some people can injest aluminum with no apparent ill effects, others suffer from a wide range of complaints, including abdominal pains, diarrhea or constipation, gas, hemorrhoids, itchy anus, duodenal ulcers, kidney and bladder problems, heart problems, itchy skin, extreme sensitivity to alcohol, thrombosis, and mental disturbances, such as an inability to make decisions.

Aluminum is a poison. If you boil water in an aluminum pot for one half hour and place the water in a glass, you will see light feathery particles floating around in the water. According to the homeopathic principle of potentization, when food or liquid is cooked in aluminum, the agitation caused by the heating process creates a potency of aluminum. This means that when a piece of pie just sits in an aluminum dish, only a small amount of aluminum can enter the pie. But food that has been cooked or water that has been boiled in an aluminum pot contains a potentized dosage of aluminum.

Try to avoid aluminum cookware. Since many hot water tanks are aluminum, it is better to use cold tap water for cooking and drinking, rather than hot tap water. Do not prepare herbal teas with aluminum pots.

Index

Ailments are printed in bold.